Back Pain:

I0417149

More Than a Symptom

A chiropractic patient's guide to health and wellness!

Dr. Patrick McCauley, D.C.
Board Certified Chiropractor

ISBN-13: 978-1514128206
ISBN-10: 1514128209

Introduction

What's the point of this book? What am I trying to say with all this information? My hope is that you get an idea of what healthcare truly is. I am hoping that you come to the realization that the current medical model is not the "be all, end all" that we have been sold. It's a great system for traumas and emergencies. It is also a good place to gather information on what it is you are dealing with so that you can decide what actions you need to take. The science behind the medical profession is not what it is all cracked up to be. Healthcare is not going to the doctors, having your blood drawn for blood work to be done so they can decide what drug you will need to be on for the rest of your life. It's not having your flu shot every year or taking over-the-counter medicines for every minor discomfort you experience only to find out after several years of this "healthcare," your kidneys are failing, or you discover that your liver is damaged and now requires surgery.

Health begins with discovering what it is you want. What are your health goals? Start by educating yourself on some of the options that are out there to help you reach your goals. Discuss your goals with your doctor. Learn from true healthcare professionals whose knowledge goes beyond drugs or surgery. The natural process of the body is that everything works together. You cannot affect one aspect of the body without affecting the whole body. Modern medicine, with their great science, has all these "specialists" who only work on one aspect of the body. This works great when an area is affected by trauma. However, breaking up every aspect of the human body into "specialties," for "healthcare" goes against nature.

One of the amazing aspects that drew me to chiropractic is that chiropractic is a natural healthcare system that looks at the body as a whole.

Chiropractic treatments are done in an effort to help the whole body. Chiropractic understands that by effecting the spine, you effect the whole body. Chiropractic also understands that there are other components to restoring ones health as explained in the Five Fundamental Keys to Health in chapter 6.

I would ask that you read this book all the way through. Do not skim over a subject because you already know something about it. The words "I already know that" can literally cause you harm. If your mind believes that you know about a particular subject, then your mind will prevent you from allowing any new information in. So I ask you to read the entire book with an open mind. Once the information is in there, then you can decide if it is useful or not. I'm also going to suggest that you study up on the Five Fundamental Keys to Health. It may take a few minutes out of your busy schedule, but I believe it will be worth it. People who won't take the time to improve their health will have to take the time for their illness. Make some changes to your eating habits, your exercise routine, your thinking, and get your spine checked. Remember you do not have to make huge changes. Make minor changes as you progress along in this new healthy lifestyle. Growing old should not consist of doctor visit after doctor visit or pill after pill. Know this: You and your body can perform great feats, and you are both truly amazing!

Effort has nothing to do with anyone else! You control effort.

Yours in Health,

Patrick McCauley, D.C.

Table of Contents

Chapter 1
A Typical Story

Never mind what you have done in the past.
What are you going to do from this point on?

It is disturbing to me but the truth is, a typical patient usually doesn't enter a chiropractic office until he or she has tried several other practitioners. These would include a general practitioner, orthopedic surgeon, a physical 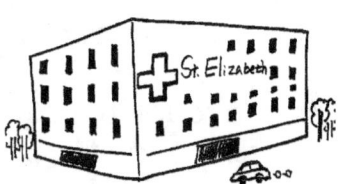 therapist and maybe receiving a massage or two. After those efforts have yielded little or no results, the patient may decide to seek chiropractic care. This appears to be the way the current medical model works. But this model is a very costly program, both financially and physically. Delaying proper treatment may allow a condition to get worse. Let's imagine how a typical patient deals with what seems to be simple low back pain that suddenly came on after he bent over to pick up his 2-year-old son.

Joe is home on the weekend playing with his son. Joe begins to pick up his son. He instantly hears a "pop" and 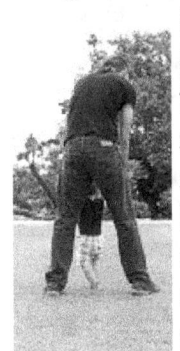 begins to feel lower back pain. He gingerly works his way to the couch to rest; but as time goes on, the pain begins to get worse. He decides to take some over-the-counter meds (OTCs), but they seem to provide little help; and he realizes that he is done for the day. A neighbor friend stops by and notices the discomfort Joe is in and offers some prescription pain killers from a recent knee surgery. Joe decides to give them a try.

Needless to say, this can be very dangerous. As the pain continues to worsen, Joe isn't sure what to do. Should he ice it? Should he place a heating pack on it?

After a few hours goes by, he has exhausted all his options and there is no improvement. In fact, it seems to be getting worse. His wife, who at this point is concerned, calls the on-call emergency nurse. The nurse advises him to take some muscle relaxers and/or an anti-inflammatory. She may also advise heat or some ice and rest. Not much help there.

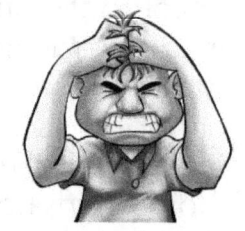

After a rough night of not being able to get any sleep, Joe tries to get out of bed. In an attempt to get upright, he notices that not only has his back pain increased overnight, but he has developed additional pain that is now running down the back of his leg. This pain is preventing him from walking normally. After one look at Joe, his wife decides it is time to go to the emergency room. After several hours and a few tests later, the doctor tells him that there were no significant findings and gives him much of the same advice received from the on- call nurse from the night before. Only this time, he is given stronger medications. Even though the visit didn't result in much help, Joe seems to feel better, knowing it wasn't some form of cancer or major pathology. Like most of the population, Joe has had occasional back pains before, but nothing like this!

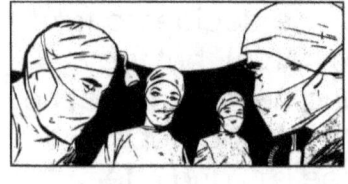

A couple of days later Joe has only improved slightly, so he decides to go see his primary care physician. Showing some concern for Joe's condition, the primary care physician begins to perform additional tests by drawing some blood and ordering an MRI.

After a few days of rest and still no improvement, Joe returns to his primary care physician for his MRI results. He is told he has a moderate disc bulge, and his doctor prescribes stronger medications, refers him to physical therapy and offers a referral to an orthopedic surgeon. During his visit to the orthopedic surgeon, the doctor suggests that they perform spinal surgery to repair the bulging disc.

Not too excited about the idea of doing spinal surgery, Joe elects to hold off on surgery and decides to try physical therapy for a few weeks first.

A note here: Be careful of the "disc bulge" diagnosis. There have been studies done where 100 people were taken off the streets, who had no pain, had an MRI and nearly half of those had a diagnosis of a "disc bulge." Although MRIs are helpful, they are not definitive.

After a few weeks of physical therapy, Joe's condition improved slightly. He can at least go back to work, although on a limited work schedule. As his frustration begins to escalate, he sees his doctor again. At this point the doctor suggests a cortisone shot to ease the pain. Joe agrees to the injection into his spine, regardless of potential harm due to the possible side-effects.

Frankly, when most people are in pain for months and their finances are being affected causing a drastic reduction in their quality of life, they are willing to accept almost anything without asking a lot of questions if they believe it will help.

In my experience with my patients receiving cortisone shots as well as having discussions with medical doctors, cortisone can be a hit or miss. Some people respond well and the pain goes away.

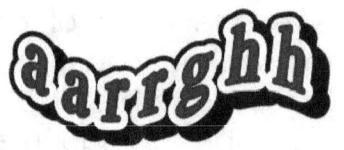

But some people receive no relief at all. Occasionally, a patient may get worse, not to mention the potential damage it may cause. There is a reason they typically will only give three injections to an area. For Joe's case, let's say the shots seem to help a bit, but the pain down the leg persists. He makes yet another appointment to see his primary care physician, which results in a referral to the neurologist. The neurologist performs his examination and then has Joe come back for a nerve conduction test.

When Joe returns to do the test, he receives an alarming shock to his leg that makes him jump right out of his seat. At this point, he has had enough and is not willing to continue with the testing.

A few months have gone by with many visits to his doctor, physical therapist and specialists. He is still in considerable pain and has no real solutions or answers. Joe has been taking several different medications to relieve his pain and even some to help him sleep. He is frustrated, angry and, frankly, scared. Noticing Joe's pain, a friend suggests he go see a chiropractor. Joe is hesitant at first, but after some strong persuasion from his wife, he decides to make an appointment for an evaluation and consultation.

All progress is due to those who were not satisfied to let well enough alone.

Chapter 2

The Chiropractic Visit

INSIDE-OUT CONCEPT

Anyone can say they care, but not everyone can prove it.

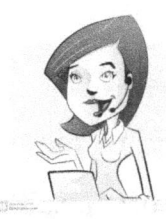

Upon entering the chiropractic office, Joe noticed that the office setting was much less sterile than most doctor's offices. In fact, it seemed very pleasant. The receptionist even knew who he was. "You must be Joe. Welcome to our office. I'm Lisa. It is very nice to meet you." Joe already started to feel less nervous about his visit; after all, he has heard a few "things" about chiropractors. Things like they are a little quaky and they try to make you go forever.

After the paperwork was finished, Joe was sent back to see the doctor immediately. A few minutes later the doctor entered the room. After a quick introduction, the doctor began his consultation. The doctor was very thorough with his questions, and he seemed genuinely concerned about Joe's overall health as opposed to just his back pain. He wanted to know how this condition has affected Joe with the things that he liked to do, his daily activities, like playing with his son or working in the garden. Every other doctor was only concerned about the pain. No other doctor cared about how it was affecting Joe in his personal life. This was refreshing; and Joe began to really pay attention to him.

After the consultation, the doctor took Joe to the exam room and began performing his physical exam.

It was the most comprehensive evaluation Joe had received. The doctor explained what he was doing and why he was doing it. Joe finally felt like he was being listened to and cared for.

After the comprehensive exam, the doctor had informed Joe that he would need some time to review all his notes and the medical records, x-rays and MRI that Joe had brought into the office.

The doctor explained to Joe that once he reviewed all the records, he would be prepared to give Joe a report of findings. In the report of findings he will let Joe know if, in fact, he is a chiropractic candidate. If so, he will be prepared to give his recommendations of care. If he discovers that he is not a chiropractic candidate, he will be prepared to refer him to the appropriate doctor or specialist. Either way the doctor was determined to make some progress in Joe's condition. Joe felt like he made the right decision and was 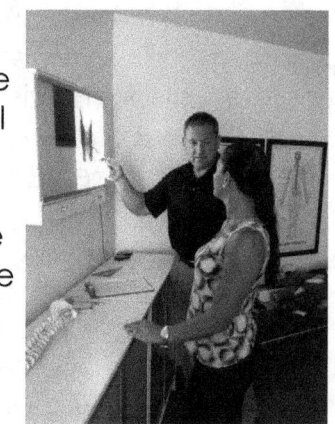 hopeful the chiropractor could help. Joe scheduled his report of findings for the very next day.

Report of Findings:

Joe was a little nervous as he did not know what to expect. The doctor came in and began to review his findings. The doctor explained that based on his evaluation and findings, he believed Joe is, in fact, a chiropractic candidate.

The doctor explained that he believed he would be able to help and gave his recommendations of care. The doctor also explained in detail the course of care and how he expected the care to progress as it went along. One thing the doctor made clear was that this was a partnership and that Joe was to participate and perform the recommended exercises and stay on track with his care if he was to receive the desired results. Joe enthusiastically agreed.

Prior to Joe's first adjustment the doctor had explained exactly what he was going to do and why he felt this would help Joe's condition. Joe felt that everything the doctor was telling him made a lot of sense and at this point trusted the doctor's judgment.

The first adjustment was wild to say the least. Joe had never heard his body make cracking noises like that before. He seemed to feel just a little less tight; a sense of relief already. Joe was encouraged. After several visits Joe began to notice some significant improvements. He was moving better and had a lot less pain.

It was at this point that the doctor began implementing Joe's home exercise program, which primarily consisted of a daily stretch routine. Once the patient is near pain free and has improved in range of motion A more aggressive exercise program will be implemented.

After a couple of months, Joe was significantly improved and is beginning to get back to his normal activities. Through the course of care, Joe has learned how to better take care of himself.

11

Joe also understands what to do in the event he does have a flare-up.

Overall, Joe is very pleased that he finally went to see the chiropractor and is now telling others who are not improving or do not want to take medications to go see the chiropractor.

Summary:

The reality of this story is very similar to many visits that occur in my practice. By spending time with our patients we have the opportunity to get to the cause of the problem rather then just masking the pain. The repetition of visits allows us to remove the irritations and allow the body to recover. It also allows us to make corrections along the way as we implement stretches and exercises to restore strength, stability and flexibility to the region. You simply cannot do all that with medications.

"All things are possible until they are proven impossible-even the impossible may only be so as of now."
-Pearl Buck

Chapter 3

Current Medical Model

OUTSIDE-IN CONCEPT

You must be the change you wish to see in the world.
–Mahatma Gandhi

Back when healthcare began, there were all these remedies that claimed to "cure" all things. This is why the FDA was established; to protect the people from erroneous claims and possible harm from those infamous elixirs. The pharmaceutical companies were working hard to develop medicine to help people recover from an illness or prevent some serious disease. The medical doctors actually cared about the well-being of their patients. In fact, they would care for their patients for many years, watch their children grow up to adults and then take care of their children. When a new vaccine or a new drug was introduced, a medical doctor would literally take the time to review the scientific literature to determine if, in fact, this drug would benefit their patient. Reviewing the literature helped the doctor make an informed decision on whether the benefits of taking the drug outweighed the potential harm the drug may cause.

This is a far cry from what is going on today!

Lets take a look at "Modern Healthcare"

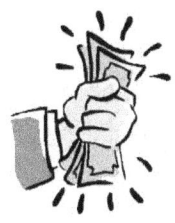 Today when you go to the medical doctor's office. there are basically only two things a medical doctor can offer you: It is either drugs or surgery. That is really it!

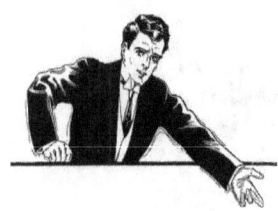 Medical schooling basically consists of training a person to discover the pathology, come up with a definitive diagnosis and, if surgery is not required, then prescribe the appropriate medication.

So in essence they do not "cure" anything. Today's healthcare is **big business.**

The doctor no longer takes the time to review the technical information on a new drug. The appropriate medication to give is usually introduced to the medical doctor by the sales representative, who typically has no medical degree or background. While the sales rep is educating the doctor on the new drug, a commercial is educating the patient on what new drug to ask for. What a perfect set up.

During my workshops we go into depth on how the current healthcare system is less than optimal in doing its job. The healthcare system is extraordinarily expensive, plagued with errors and illusions of a cure. It is estimated that Americans make up about 4% of the total world population, yet 50% of all the money in the world is spent on American medical care. It is currently the number one reason for bankruptcies in the United States. With that kind of financial resource, you would think that Americans are one of the healthiest countries in the world. According to the World Health Organization, the United States is ranked a dismal 37th among the world's health systems. The media tells us of all these medical breakthroughs in modern medicine and new high-tech equipment.

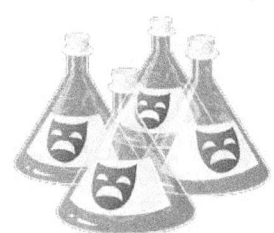 There are numerous "awareness" groups collecting substantial funds to help "cure" some type of disease, yet every year the death toll of nearly all major diseases continues to rise.

It's a fact that more and more people are dying each year from heart disease, cancer and diabetes. It appears that the current medical model just isn't working. Being cured must mean you are on your meds for life. This allopathic model of an outside-in concept is extremely expensive, shockingly ineffective and saturated with side effects, contraindications, doctor induced ailments, premature deaths and too many unnecessary procedures.

With the development of HMOs it seems that the protocols dictate what you get rather than what you need! Based on these disturbing facts, something needs to change. We need to look at what we call "healthcare" from a different perspective; a paradigm shift, if you will. We need to empower people rather than render them helpless. You MUST be more involved in your healthcare. The very concept of taking a doctor prescribed poison to mask a symptom with the misguided belief that the problem is fixed or "cured" is ignorant and irresponsible and goes against the very nature of health.

Each person is born with an innate intelligence whose sole purpose in life is to maintain balance in the body in an effort to promote health. So "healthcare" should have something to do with supporting this intelligence rather than giving it more work to do. This intelligence can perform miracles if allowed to do so.

Here are some more alarming facts.

It is estimated that the correct treatment is given less than 60% of the time; and that is based on the AMA and their own standards. I would guess it is much lower.

The current American healthcare system is the third leading cause of preventable deaths, just behind heart disease and cancer. This accounts for nearly 210,000 Americans. The whole concept of "healthcare" is based on the premise that the doctors, scientists and chemists know more about the human body than the body itself. Giving the body some foreign, harmful substance to correct what the "experts" perceive that the body is doing wrong or remove a body part that appears damaged or deemed "not necessary" is the very definition of an outside -in concept . If you have an upset stomach, take this. If you have a fever, you take that. If you have a cough, take this. It is all about taking a product to help you remove a symptom so that you feel better. That's a cure?

The flooding of clever marketing has taught us how to be great little medicine taking patients. This all starts out when we are young. The minute you are born you are injected with toxic chemicals from a vaccine to "protect" you. Marketing tells us that for every symptom there is a cure" (product) to take. "Just ask your doctor." The mere fact that the drug companies are even allowed to do commercials is beyond me. Why would they need to market to you what you need?

Let's take a look at a typical drug commercial. The commercial goes something like this: It begins with an individual who is very unhappy with their ailment.

16

They are either dealing with some pain or possibly an embarrassing issue. The story begins with the characters tugging on your emotions. As the commercial progresses you begin to feel that there is hope, that there is this miracle cure. The individual begins to show their new found happiness and freedom. They are cured and life is fabulous.

"Side-Effects"

But then as you are watching the joy on their faces, wanting the same thing, the narrator begins the disclaimer. Results may vary and some individuals have suffered the following "side-effects." One of the "side-effects' is even death but you don't care; you want to feel just like the person on the commercial. Why should anyone take a medication that has the remote possibility of death? Just as the commercial is about to end the narrator directs you to tell your doctor you want such and such drug. **You** should not be telling the doctor what drug you want. Your physician should know what you need.

How a drug that is designed to remove skin lesions, with the remote possibility of death, can be approved by the great protective FDA is another issue that is beyond me. That will be the subject of my next book. I wanted to take a moment to discuss this whole concept of "side-effects." First let me start out by saying, in reality **there is no such thing**! There is no such thing as a "side-effect." There are only effects. There are desired effects and undesirable effects. That's it. Do you know what the difference between effect and "side-effect" is?

It's Marketing.

Here are a couple of examples: Did you know that Post-It notes were developed out of a complete failure? The developer was trying to make the strongest glue possible; in his failure, he discovered another use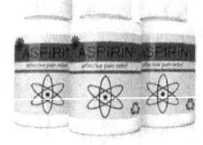

The same goes for a very popular drug. During the human testing trials, this drug was not performing as planned, and they had to stop the research. When the male subjects were reluctant to return the medications, they discovered a whole new use for this drug. So what at first was a side-effect, is now being marketed as the desired effect. And now you have a multi-billion dollar drug full of other effects. The challenge is that this botched research is passed off as science. And that science affects your health. In a later chapter we will go into more detail on how a drug gets to market so you understand what the "gold standard" of research is for allowing a drug to reach the market and your body. It's not what it is all cracked up to be. It is also concerning as to how the drug companies, who are obligated and legally responsible, inform you of the possible side-effects. If you have received a prescription or have seen an ad for a drug, you have seen or heard the disclaimer or list of possible side-effects.

The printed version resembles a very fine-printed contract with too much information for anyone to read. The effects with the drug are hidden in plain sight, basically. The more appropriate method would be to simply list the top five most prevalent side effects in clear, easy to read, large print. However, that would not be very beneficial for marketing and may actually reduce sales.

A very valuable tool that I use on a regular basis in my office is a website called **drugs.com.** On this site you get a clear idea of what that prescription drug is all about. If you are taking medications and are not very clear on their side effects, I urge you to look them up on drugs.com.

When taking any medications, it is important to be clear on what they are and why you are taking them. Then you need to decide if the benefits outweigh the harm these drugs may cause. ***You do realize that it is your choice; right?***

Far too many people take medications without fully understanding the ramifications and that they can actually choose whether or not they want to take them.

If we are to believe that all we need to do is take a pill to fix what is ailing us, then why do we need to make any changes? The next question is if this process works, then why are more and more people dying from heart disease, cancer and diabetes every year?

The following page contains a humorous account of a typical life cycle of an American in our modern healthcare system. It is called

"The Great American Death Ceremony."

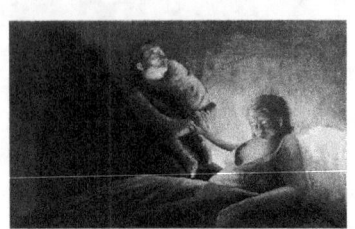

The Great American Death Ceremony

The Death Ceremony began as a crude ritual back in the days of witchcraft. In recent years, it has developed into a science. It usually takes 10-15 years; however, modern scientific advancements are shortening this period of time.

It starts with one simple aspirin for a simple headache. When one aspirin will no longer cover up the headache, take two. After a few months, when two aspirins no longer cover up the headache, you take one of the stronger compounds. By this time, it becomes necessary to take something for the ulcers, which have been caused by the aspirin.

Now that you are taking two medicines, you think you have a good start. After a few months, these medicines will begin to disrupt your liver function. If an infection develops, you will now take some penicillin. Of course, the penicillin will damage your red blood corpuscles and spleen so that you develop anemia. By this time, all of these medications will put such a strain on your kidneys that they begin to shut down.

It is now time to take more antibiotics. When these antibiotics destroy your natural resistance to disease, you can expect a general flare-up in all your systems. The next step is to cover up all of those symptoms with sulfa drugs. When your kidneys finally plug up, you can have them drained. Some poisons will build up in your system, but you can keep going quite a while this way.

By now, the medications will be so confused they won't know what they are supposed to be doing, but it doesn't really matter. If you have followed every step as directed, you can now make an appointment with your undertaker.

Practically all Americans, except for a few ignorant souls who follow nature, play this game.

From the Journal of the Certified Natural Health Professional.

Let's take a look at our seniors. It is estimated that the average American senior citizen is on 6-7 different medications or more. I've personally had a few patients who were prescribed over 12 different medications. If you practice this type of "healthcare" by following the doctor's orders, who ultimately pays the price? **You do!** I would suggest you take a more involved interest in YOUR health by gathering as much information as you can on whether there are other options. Learn about what changes you can make, and what exactly you are about to put into your body. Be informed rather than just following orders.

Another clever marketing tool is to make you believe that your condition is out of your hands. If they could get you to believe that your condition is "genetic," then there is truly nothing you can do; right? This subject is another whole book, but let me just say that true genetic conditions are few and far between. There is a difference between genetic predisposition to a condition and genetic expression of that condition. The outside-in concept disempowers us, turning us in to lifetime "healthcare" patients so by the time you are 60, you are on several medications leading a "healthy" lifestyle. This is all smoke and mirrors bringing me to my final point.

All this science and technology, years of research and manpower to develop a miracle pill to cure you of your disease sounds amazing. Did you know that in the final stages of research this breakthrough in science has to simply outperform a placebo? That's even after a carefully selected study group is put together in an effort to help the researched drug perform better, the placebo, which is usually a sugar pill, frequently performs nearly as well as the expensive drug.

The sugar pill actually cures people of their ailment nearly as often as this expensive high tech drug. Why do you think placebos are illegal now?

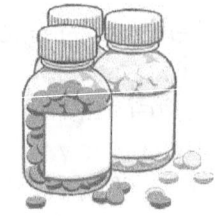

They do no harm and there are no side-effects. The sad thing is that this is the **Gold Standard**, the best we have. That to me seems to be seriously lacking, to say the least. **That is what we are calling science?**

It wasn't long ago that a doctor could actually prescribe a sugar pill then report that many of these people had a complete recovery. The mere fact that the placebo usually performs just as well as most scientifically developed drugs, should shed some light on the way the human body heals itself through the mind-body connection. The very thought that a person was taking a pill to cure them of their ailment created real biochemical changes that were essential for combating their disease. We will discuss the mind-body equation in a later chapter.

Another concern is that over-the-counter medicines are taken too lightly. Take aspirin for example. Aspirin is very common and some experts believe it to be one of the most harmless of all drugs. It is even suggested that you take aspirin as a preventative measure. Even healthy people are taking this drug. However, aspirin requires some considerable care. Even a minimal dose can cause internal bleeding and over 100,000 people die every year from aspirin alone. I read somewhere that if aspirin were to be released on the market today, it would be by prescription only. It is widely believed that aspirin was beneficial for arthritis.

However, some experts suggest that aspirin impairs the clotting function of platelets, disc-shaped substances in the blood, making it harmful in the treatment of collagen illnesses such as arthritis.

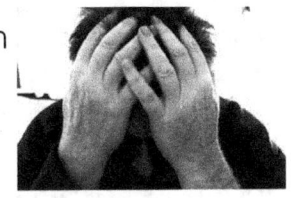

In fact, experts still cannot agree on how aspirin actually works.

THEY DON"T KNOW!!!

Look, history has been plagued with what was known as the state-of-the-art treatments or potions only to find out later that that initial treatment was actually harmful.

The FDA was originally formed to protect the people from harm. With the growing number of deaths and illness due to FDA approved drugs, this protection appears to have faded.

Let's take blood letting for example. This practice was used for centuries and was believed to be essential for rapid recovery. Only later, doctors discovered it was actually weakening the patient. This practice is believed to have contributed to George Washington's death. I believe several common practices today will be deemed harmful in the near future. Vaccines and chemo therapy are already being suggested but are being dismissed.

One of the most glaring weaknesses that still exist today is the healthcare system's failure to recognize the significant value of nutrition. Just look at their meals. In 1969 the White House Conference on Food, Nutrition and Health noted that the great failure of medical schools is that they pay minimal attention to the science of nutrition. That was 45 years ago and yet even today nutrition is still not a course in the medical colleges.

And finally, the hospitals themselves. They are consumed by multiple shortcomings with the presence of strong bacteria and numerous errors in both administration and performance. There is statistical proof that hospital deaths decrease when there is a strike involving the doctors and nurses. It would appear that the hospital is no place for the seriously ill.

Let me be clear. I do not want to seem like I am medical bashing. I believe many of our healthcare professionals care about their patients. My point here is that the current medical system is significantly flawed and that drugs are a tool to be used only when absolutely necessary. Obviously, medicine has a purpose.

There are times that medications are necessary, but a good doctor is aware of their power and the potential damage they cause. If I am ever involved in an accident and are severely injured and am in real bad shape, then give me any drug and perform any surgery you deem necessary to save my life. But, you can bet that I will be more than just a passive observer when it comes to my health and well being. I had to do this to save my mom's life when she was dealing with terminal lung cancer several years ago

I do not believe we should simply follow directions and take a drug for the rest of our life and call it healthcare. If you are going to put some form of poison in your body, you should be well-informed of all the effects and weigh in on whether or not the effects outweigh the benefits. For me, that would be a rare occasion. There are other choices.

Personally, I believe we need a paradigm shift in thinking when it comes to healthcare. In fact, we should change the name from healthcare to crisis care or acute care or relief care; something to show that this is a supportive, temporary treatment to help you get back on track.

I believe emergency room doctors perform miracles every day. My family and I do not go to the medical doctor every time we have a cough, sniffle or fever. We will discuss a bit later what health really is and how to obtain it.

" The secret of change is to focus all of your energy not on fighting the old, but on building the new"
– SOCRATES

Chapter 4

What is Health?

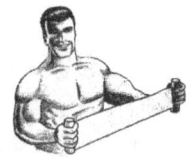

No matter how slow you go you are still passing everyone on the couch.

At my weekend workshops I ask, "What is health?" I ask the audience to help me list some answers on the board. The most common response I get is "feeling good." Obviously, feeling good is a part of health, but feeling good alone would suggest that as long as we have no symptoms, then we are healthy. Is that really true? Here are a few examples of

Feeling good
Not sick
Having energy
No pain
Being active
Eating better

everyday people who are feeling good and appear to be healthy, but, in fact, are very sick.

For example, a women could have breast cancer for years before any symptom occurs. Or a gentleman could have prostate cancer before a single symptom develops. A cavity may take some time before you feel the pain and that's a hole in your tooth. These examples appear to be Extreme; however, judging how healthy you are based on symptoms or lack of symptoms can be dangerous.

I read an article that stated that in more than 50% of the cases that involve heart attack deaths, the first symptom is death. Those people never get a second chance. Those people were symptom free up until they died. Were these people healthy? Of course not. So the mere fact that we are symptom free **does not** necessarily mean we are healthy. Wouldn't you agree? This is one of the challenges that I see with our current healthcare system.

The medical profession would like you to believe in this pain-free concept. It is evident in all their advertisements. If you are suffering from this, then take that. So once you take 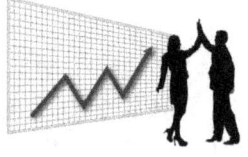 this pill and no longer have a symptom, then you must be healthy! Right? We have shown that it is not always the case.

It appears that the medical industry is very focused on the symptom and the cure. The cure involves removing the symptom. If the pharmaceutical industry can come up with a pill that can remove the symptom, then they have provided a service, not to mention the billions of dollars in profit. A great many alternative health practitioners would argue that the symptom is what guides you towards restoring your health and needs to be addressed, not simply removed. We spoke earlier about the dangers of ignoring the symptom.

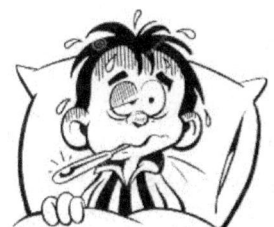 On the other side of the coin, symptoms don't always mean we are sick either. I often give a scenario in my talks of a child who appears to be what most people would label sick: the child has a high fever, vomiting and diarrhea. Not very fun! But is this child sick? Or, is the child healthy? Of course, when I ask this question to my audiences, the overwhelming response is "Yes, the child is sick." Well, let's take a look at this. Let's say the child ate something that the body perceives as harmful, like an invader such as a bacteria or a poison. The body's natural defense is to remove it, if it can or kill it. So the body begins to fight. It may have diarrhea to try to remove the invader. In an effort to kill the invader the body begins to develop a fever. The fever is part of the cellular mediated immune response. This happens for a reason.

For every degree in temperature rise in your body, the speed at which your white blood cells can travel to the invader, and thus their effectiveness, is doubled. What does that mean? That means that if you have a fever of 104 degrees, the speed at which your white blood cells can move is 64 times greater than that of the normal body temperature of 98 degrees. That's very efficient. The point is that the fever is a natural response created by the immune system in an effort to speed up its process of destroying the invader or disease.

It is not something that your body is doing wrong. The last thing you want to do is suppress the fever. This will impair the immune system and could allow the condition to worsen. Now, at this point, I am sure I have raised a few eyebrows regarding the child's temperature, as the medical profession would have you go to the emergency room at this point.

The key when dealing with the high fever is not allowing it to get any higher than 104 degrees, as brain cells began to die at 106 degrees. The other important factor is the demeanor of the child; is he lethargic, weak, and unable to keep fluids down? Or is he still wanting to play and move around? If he is lethargic, and is unable to keep fluids down, he may become dehydrated and needs to be seen right away. If he is able to play some and drink some fluids, he should be fine. Dehydration is the concern. The current medical model would have you take medications to stop the vomiting or stop the diarrhea and stop the fever. This may cause the condition to get worse. And those medications only address the symptoms, not the cause.

Not to mention the dangers of a reaction to the harmful substances in the medications themselves. I also want to mention that several other countries discourage giving a cold or flu medicine to any child under the age 14; in the United States, it is a child under 6.

I discussed the body's immune system. Let's talk about how your body functions on a day-to-day basis. The body strives for what is called **homeostasis.** Every second of every day your body is working hard to create homeostasis. Homeostasis is the body's ability to maintain a state of ease or balance.

Every day there are invaders that attempt to camp out in your body. There are cancer cells in your body that are taken care of by your immune system without you knowing about it. There are a whole host of actions your body does to defend your health, without your knowledge.

Does sickness even exist?

I know we see and hear about it every single day. The medical profession constantly informs us of how deeply concerned they are about protecting everyone from the common flu with their completely safe and effective flu shot. I'm being very sarcastic about the safe and effective part.

Let's look at it from a different perspective in this new paradigm. What if we looked at sickness as being this opportunistic thing that can only appear when a deficiency exists. I believe sickness is just like darkness.

Does darkness truly exist?

We see darkness on a daily basis; right?

Let's say you are in a room that is completely dark and you want to lighten the room up a bit. How much darkness do you need to remove to lighten up the room? The obvious answer is you cannot remove any darkness. You cannot take darkness out of the room to lighten it up. So how do you lighten up the room? You bring in light. So if you cannot remove darkness and the only way to brighten the room is to bring in light, then I ask you again: Does darkness truly exist? Well at this point you might say I understand your questioning, but I still see darkness all the time. So I would say to you, "darkness does exist." However, darkness only exists in the absence of light. If there is light, there is no darkness. What's my point?

Sickness only exists in the absence of health.

In today's medical model a person becomes sick and we want to give him or her something to remove the sickness or perform surgery to remove the seemingly diseased body part. In that scenario, we are reducing the effectiveness of the body's ability to adjust or, simply put, chasing a ghost.

Dorland's Medical Dictionary defines health as "a state of optimal physical, mental and social well being and not merely the absence of disease and infirmity." What needs to be done is to restore health in that individual. Give the body what it needs to defend itself rather than give it another poison to deal with. That's true healthcare.

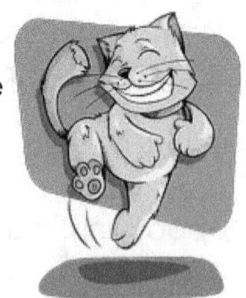

The allopathic model consists of an outside-in mentality. The science and the medical industry believes it has become smarter than the innate intelligence that has evolved over millions of years. Medicine has been around maybe 150 years. An infant by comparison.

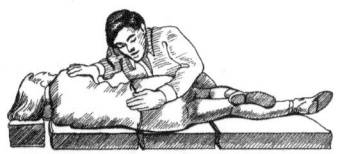

Once we begin to perform procedures that help individuals improve their health and assist the body in restoring homeostasis, then we will all be a much healthier species. As it stands now, humans are the sickest animals on the planet. One of the major challenges with this type of healthcare is that it does not yield instant results.

Removing sickness from an individual to improve his or her health is much like trying to remove darkness to brighten a room. Chiropractic tries to restore function and allow the body to begin to heal itself. I will go in depth more on how we do that later. Most of the perceived success of medicine is hiding behind the body's capacity to adapt and heal itself. In fact, we usually become better, in spite of our effort to the contrary.

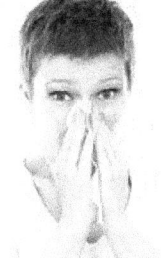

So then why do we get sick?

Why does a person who seemingly is healthy become ill? I believe that there are basically two main reasons we all become sick. We are either toxic or we are deficient. Either of these states weaken the body, allowing it to become susceptible to invaders. I can assure you one thing: You are most certainly not getting a headache because you are deficient in Aspirin.

Have you ever wondered why some people become ill and others do not when they are all exposed to the same person who is ill and contagious?

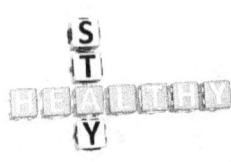 Well, some of those people must have a stronger immune system and are able to fight off the invader before any symptoms occur. Others are not so fortunate and the invader delivers a much stronger attack.

I would suggest that the people who became susceptible to the invader were either deficient or toxic, compromising their immune system. Now the next question is, how do we become toxic or deficient? I could write a whole book on that subject alone, but here are a few suggestions: poor diet, lack of exercise, movement deficiencies, lack of sleep, chronic stress, poor air quality, poor water quality and medications, to name a few. So in an effort to become healthy, we must live a healthy lifestyle that prevents us from becoming toxic or deficient. Eating a healthy diet, getting plenty of exercise , getting plenty of rest, drinking plenty of water, getting adjusted, and reducing stress are a few things we can implement to improve our health. I use the following health scale in my workshops to help people really put some thought into their own health as it is today.

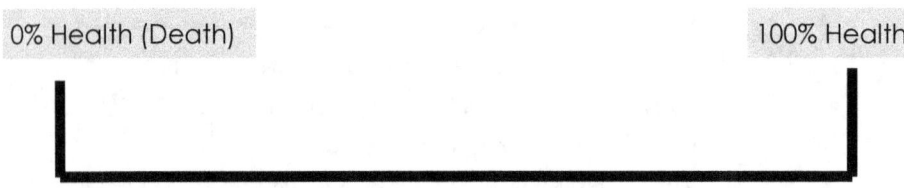

0% Health (Death)   100% Health

- Where are you on this scale?
- How do you know?
- More importantly, which direction are you heading?

Remember there is no such thing as status quo. You are either actively getting healthier, or you are getting less healthy. I encourage my patients to do something intentional towards improving their health. Some patients claim that they 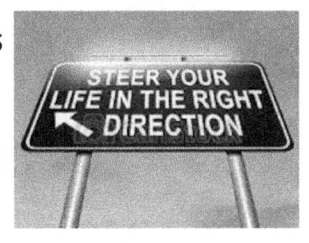 get plenty of exercise because their jobs require them to walk a lot, and they have been doing that for years. Well, if you are not intentionally doing more, then you are regressing. Your body adapts to the resistance and therefore, stops progressing. Be honest with yourself.

I do not believe the concept of healthcare through medications. There is usually a better way. Everyone was born to be healthy. I am hoping this chapter lights a fire in you to become more involved with your own health. When working with a patient, I try to help empower them to make small steps towards improving their heath for a better quality of life. I firmly believe that there is a direct correlation to health and quality of life.

Get your health back!

Chapter 5

The Effects of Stress!

Stressed is desserts spelled backwards!

I wanted to write a chapter on stress because of all the potential health issues that chronic stress is believed to be linked to. It is believed that nearly 80% of all illness can be linked to chronic stress. This would indicate that if you are able to reduce the stress, or more importantly, your response to stress, then you may be able to drastically reduce your chances of becoming ill.

Let's talk about some of the affects chronic stress has on our health. I do a health talk that primarily focuses on stress alone. We cover many aspects of health; some of which we will discuss here. Some of the major signs of stress include the following:

Headaches
Fatigue
Neck or Back Pain
Loss of Sleep
Digestive Trouble
Allergies/Sinus Trouble
Irritability, Mood Swings, Hormonal Problems

Additionally, stress doubles your risk of having a heart attack, it increases your likelihood of developing a serious illness like diabetes, E.D., and even cancer. It may also affect your relationships, your work performance and overall health, which greatly affect a persons quality of life.

How can stress do all that?

Before we talk about what is going on in our bodies during stress, let's talk about why our bodies reacts the way it does to a stressful situation. Why would the body do something that is bad for us?

STRESS

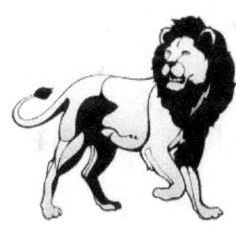 Stress is what is affectionately called the "fight or flight" response. We have all felt it. That sudden flinch causing our muscle to quickly flex, that burst of adrenaline and an increase in heart rate along with a whole host of other reactions. Believe it or not, this process is designed to save your life! These reactions are designed to help you prepare to fight or run for your life.

Let's look at a lion and gazelle. A lion sneaks up on its meal hiding in the brush. As he gets closer he begins to prepare for the opportunity to leap. However, at the last second, the gazelle sees the lion and begins to run for its life. The chase is on! Every step these animals are using every bit of energy and strength to either get a meal or to avoid being a meal. Every single muscle fiber is being used, heart rates are elevated to supply the necessary tissues with the proper fuel and oxygen. Boom, boom, boom, the intense pounding of every step. A few minutes into the chase, the lion begins to get closer. But the lion knows he cannot keep this up much longer, so he takes a shot and leaps at the gazelle. But the gazelle leaps to the right at that precise moment and gets away. The chase is over.

The lion begins to walk back towards its pride as it cools down. The gazelle looks for a peaceful spot to graze. Within 10 minutes, both animals are as they were prior to the chase.

This is a far cry from what we do. First of all, we are rarely in a true life or death situation. What typically happens, especially in the Bay Area, is a small situation occurs while we are already in a heighted state. An example would be what happens nearly 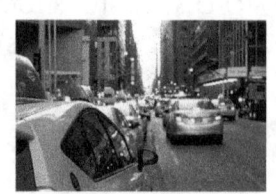 everyday on our highways. We begin our morning by hitting the snooze button one too many times. Now we really need to get going. We are getting dressed and falling behind. We hastily grab our coffee as we are heading out the door, and we spill some coffee on our shirt. No time to change as we race out the door.

Of course today there is a bit more traffic, so we begin to get a little anxious knowing that we might be late for that meeting. Then it happens, someone aggressively cuts us off 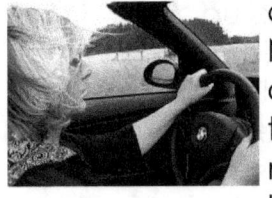 causing us to actually slam on our brakes. Now our heart rate is way up! Now we are a bit upset, and we need to let them know that we disapprove of their driving methods. Our desire to show this person how wronged we were is getting strong. We are having a difficult time getting next to them, depriving us of expressing our displeasure. This process of attempting to get next to them goes on for a few minutes. Then we finally see an opportunity to give them a piece of our mind. As we get next to them, they swiftly take the next exit never to be seen again. Now we feel even more wronged because we have unfinished business and believe they probably did it on purpose knowing we were trying to let him know they were wrong.

Now, the only way to let out our frustrations is to share this experience with several of our coworkers. And every time we bring it up, we get to relive the experience, while getting all tensed up again. This is just one example. I could have easily told a story about a coworker, a boss, a family member or a friend. And some people experience several of these on a daily basis. No wonder everyone is stressed out!

What's the difference between the wild animal and the human animal? First of all, this really wasn't a life or death situation. Second of all, we never had a chance to burn off all those chemicals that were released when the "fight or flight" response occurred. Finally, we carried this episode with us all day, each time releasing more chemicals and never really burning them off. I don't imagine that the gazelle returned to his heard telling everyone about how he was nearly eaten by a lion. Nor does the lion return to his pride complaining about the one that got away. They simply relax and let it go!

So let's take a look at what goes on during a "fight or flight" episode. First of all, there are a whole host of chemical reactions that happen in the body as you are in a heightened state. We are going to touch on a few that seem to be contributing to some of the health issues we deal with every day.

On the following page there is a diagram illustrating a few of the reactions the body performs when in a heightened state:

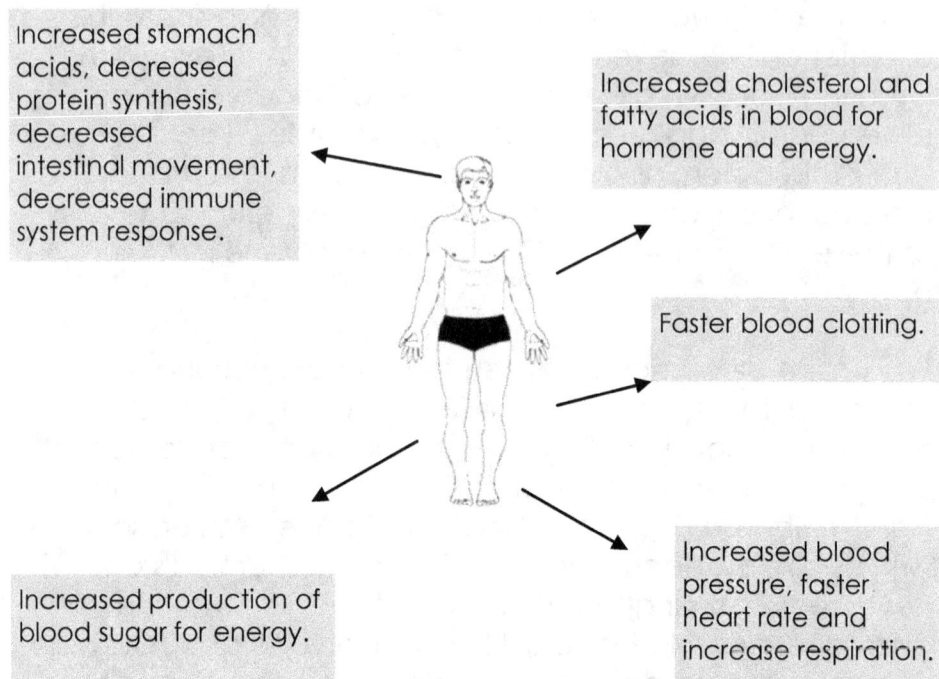

Increased stomach acids, decreased protein synthesis, decreased intestinal movement, decreased immune system response.

Increased cholesterol and fatty acids in blood for hormone and energy.

Faster blood clotting.

Increased production of blood sugar for energy.

Increased blood pressure, faster heart rate and increase respiration.

So now you can see how chronic stress can affect your health. So when you are not feeling well and you go to the doctor, it creates more stress. They tell you you have high blood pressure, high cholesterol, and you are pre diabetic. Well, no wonder. So it is important for you to recognize when you are in a stressful state and do your best to remove the stress. I have put a few ideas on how you can do that on the next few pages .

Dear stress,
I am breaking up with you.

WAYS TO REDUCE YOUR STRESS

Avoid the stress:
Learn to say "NO"

Get to know your limits and try not to overextend yourself. You must refuse to accept added responsibilities in both your professional and personal life. By taking on more than you can handle, you are creating a chronic stressful situation for yourself.

To-do list

Most of us have a to-do list that is too large. We need to reduce our to-do lists. Ideally, you would create a master list of things to do and on a daily basis, take the top six most important tasks and handle those to completion. Of course, there are always things that come up, so leave some time in your schedule for those things.

Alter the situation
Bring your "A" game

Don't cruise and give half effort. Deal with things head on and give full effort. Don't allow for distractions. By taking control of your actions, you are in the driver's seat of your life.

Manage your time

A lot of stress can develop because of poor time management, causing you to get behind. Being stretched too thin makes it difficult to stay calm and think clearly. Once you create a to-do list with your top six projects, put an amount of time you are able to give to each project;

and remembering to leave some floating time for emergencies.

Adjust to the stress

Think big

Put the stressful situation in perspective. Most of the time, no matter how bad we think it is at the moment, we usually look back and laugh at what we once thought was so detrimental. Will this really matter a month from now or a year from now? Probably not.

Perfection vs. excellence

Striving for perfection can cause a tremendous amount of stress. This puts an unrealistic pressure on yourself. Try striving for excellence. Do your best. After all, that is all you can do, which usually works out fine.

Be grateful

When stress is weighing on you take a moment to think about all the things that you are grateful for, especially your own attributes. You are truly one of a kind.

"Stress is the trash of modern life – we all generate it but if you don't dispose of it properly, it will pile up and over-take your life."

– Danzae Pace

Some things you just can't control

Accept the things you cannot change

There are things in life you can't do anything about. Do not stress over those. Direct your efforts on the things you can do something about.

Stay positive

When facing some challenging moments, you should focus on a couple of concepts. First, look for the silver lining; it is always there. Secondly, do what Steve Jobs did. When dealing with some difficult challenges, he would always say to himself "know that the dots will connect."

Forgive

When we hang on to anger and resentment for the actions of others, this creates a lot of stress for us and holds us back. Learn to forgive those who we feel have hurt us in some way. The holding on to resentment and anger is only hurting ourselves.

Some helpful tips on how to relax and recharge

- Spend a few moments outdoors
- Have a good workout
- Take a long bath
- Play with a pet
- Get a massage
- Listen to your favorite music
- Work in your garden
- Savor a good coffee or tea
- Write in your journal
- Read a good book
- Go for a walk
- Watch something funny

Chapter 6

Fundamental Keys To Health

Because today is another chance to get it right.

When a new patient commits to care in my office, I strongly suggest that they attend my Spinal Care class. The reason this class is so important is it gives me a chance to really educate a person on what it is we do and why it is important for them. I also get a 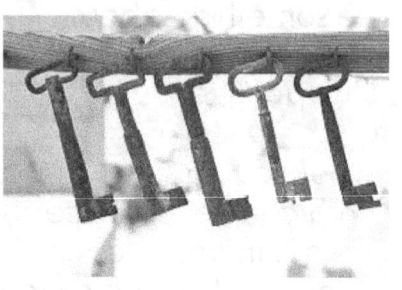 chance to get to know my patients on a more casual basis, outside the treatment room. One of the topics we discuss in this class is called The Fundamental Keys to Health. The reason I have this topic in a spinal care class is that I believe that with the overwhelming amount of information on the internet today, trying to decide what to believe in and what to do can be a daunting task, to say the least. One expert may say you need do this to be healthy. The next expert will tell you that if you do that, you will die. The really scary part is that they both have compelling reasons why their concept is true. So in this class I break down the fundamental keys to health, making it simple and easy to implement.

One of the challenges I see with my patients when trying to make some changes to their health is that they are so overwhelmed that that never start anything. When implementing anything in my office, whether it is treatment, a new exercise routine or some daily stretches, I encourage my patients to take baby steps. Create the proper habit for the long haul not for the quick fix. Quick fixes are rarely a fix at all; they are simply a band-aid. Small steps over a lengthy period of time can make a huge difference.

It seems that everyone wants instant results. Regardless of the task, we want to reach our goal now. If we want to lose weight, we want it as fast as possible; so we do a crash diet. Or we want to finally get in shape, so we usually go all out in the beginning then quickly burn out.

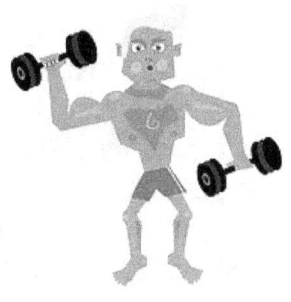

If we are in pain, we want instant relief without any reflection on what might be the cause of our pain. This practice does not work and, in fact, can be very harmful. Crash diets usually leaves a person worse off than when they started, becoming heavier than when they began. The inability to stick with an exercise routine is not healthy either; we already talked about some of the ramifications of not addressing the cause of your pain. So the key is baby steps done consistently to make some real changes.

I have several patients that seem to have the same New Year's resolutions year in and year out: Either lose weight or begin an exercise program. After just a few weeks, they begin to fade. And less than a couple of months later, they are completely off track. I see it every year at the gym. The gym gets a bit crowded for the first couple of weeks then people begin to drop off. Within a month, it's back to the normal group. I believe that they tried to do too much. It is difficult to all of a sudden put aside a couple of hours per

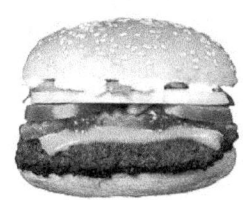

day to do a new task in your already busy schedule. The enthusiasm keeps you going for a month or so but quickly fades. Not to mention that results do not occur fast enough to fuel this new found enthusiasm. Baby steps is the key.

I put on a workshop called The 3 Biggest Mistakes Most People Make When In Pain, where we discuss this concept of a 1 degree shift in detail. This simple concept helps people make real changes.

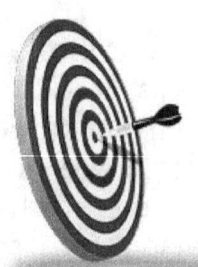

Just 1 degree of change done over a year's time can make a **huge** difference. Look, most people are practicing this concept already, by making poor diet choices, eating fast food every now and then, eating a bit too much food every now and then, maybe a few too many desserts. Then bam, all of a sudden it's 10 years later they are 50 pounds heavier. Let's make a small change for the better to create a huge and lasting difference.

So as we go through the fundamental keys to health, think about some of the small changes you could make in each area. Sustain these changes for a lengthy period of time and watch the changes occur. Following is what I believe to be The Five Fundamental Keys to Health and, more importantly, towards a better quality of life.

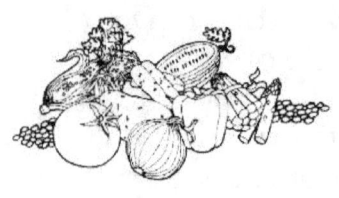

I assume most people who are on their death bed would gladly give any possession or money away for better health and more time. So while under my care, we implement simple procedures to help a person not only to get out of pain, but improve their overall health for a better quality of life. An example of this would be the daily stretch routine supplied in this book.

So the Fundamental Keys to Health consist of information as to why you should make a change and simple tips on how to make the change.

There are basically five fundamental keys that I believe would support a healthy lifestyle.

In my office it's not just about pain, it's about developing a quality of life. I believe there is a direct correlation between health and quality of life.

Fundamental Key # 1

Proper food, or more precisely, proper nutrients. The bottom line: What we eat and drink is fuel for the body. You truly are what you eat. Everything you put into the tank, so to speak, is broken down and delivered to the various departments. If the product you put into the tank is of poor quality, then the results you will get will be less than optimal. This means the immune system will function less than optimally, your digestion and energy will be less than optimal, and your thinking and rest will be less than optimal. Nutrients affect the whole system. Proper nutrients provide the body with the proper tools to allow you to function with more energy, have less body fat, have better brain function, improve cardiac health and so on.

Proper nutrients will assist your body in fending off diseases

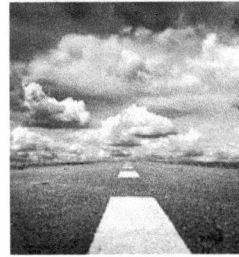

like, diabetes, heart disease and even cancer, to name a few. There is not one system in your body that would not improve with better nutrients. Proper nutrition is not about losing body fat. It is about supplying the body what it needs to function at an optimal level.

It is no different than a well run company. Every department in that company has a specific function. As long as that department has all the support and supplies it needs to do its job efficiently, then everything is working at an optimal level. If you deprive a department of some of its support or supplies that are necessary, then that department begins to break down, thus, the whole company begins to function less than optimally. Would this company close down in a week or two? Probably not, but if the problem is not addressed over time, it may have a detrimental effect on the whole company.

So eating that fast food meal every now and then isn't going to shut you down right away, but over time the effects begin to show. Blood pressure begins to rise, cholesterol levels begin to rise, energy begins to decrease; and suddenly, years later, you are now on several medications wondering what happened. "I used to be so young and full of energy" is what I often hear. Don't let this be you. Begin to make some changes in what you put in that valuable body of yours. Say no to fast food and have desserts only once in while. Reduce your alcohol. I'm not saying completely stop it all. But I believe we all can make a few changes that could drastically improve our overall health. Add a few healthy habits to your life. Once you begin to make a few changes in what you put in your body, the way you feel will begin to change.   It is a journey worth taking.

The following pages contain some healthy food choices and a bit of information as to why these are good for you. You can start with these as you begin this new path.

It is health that is real wealth and not pieces of gold and silver.

-Mahatma Gandhi

Key Healthy Foods

HEALTHY GREENS: Contain folate, calcium and other nutrients that support bone health, protect against cognitive decline, and help prevent age-related eye problems. Diets high in cruciferous veggies, such as broccoli and cabbage, help reduce risk of memory loss and cancer.

BERRIES: Blueberries, blackberries, and cranberries are rich in antioxidant compound known as anthocyanins, which have been known to slow the growth of certain cancer cells as well as improve brain function, muscle tone, and balance.

OLIVE OIL: Rich in antioxidants and anti-inflammatory monounsaturated fats, olive oil figures prominently in the Mediterranean diet. It may explain the lower rates of cardiovascular disease, cancer, and age-related cognitive decline in people who follow this way of eating.

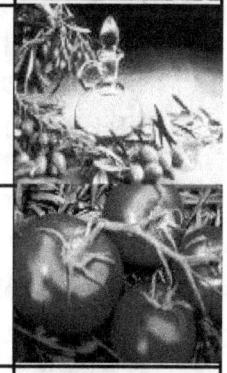

TOMATOES: Certain red fruits, including tomatoes, contain lycopene, an antioxidant compound that helps maintain youthful skin texture and may reduce the risk of some types of cancer (especially prostate, lung, and stomach cancers) as well as heart disease.

NUTS: Varieties such as almonds and walnuts contain a generous helping of healthy fats, vitamins, and protein that benefit cardiovascular and brain health. Nuts are also high in compounds that ease inflammation.

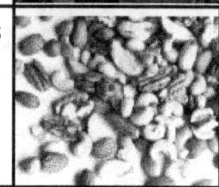

RED GRAPES: Grapes offer an antioxidant called resveratrol that's been shown to extend the life of lab animals. Resveratrol has anti-inflammatory and anticoagulant properties, which may explain why red wine and purple grape juice also help promote heart health.

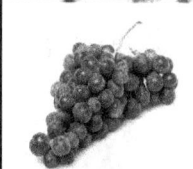

FISH: An important part of the Japanese and Mediterranean diet, oily fish provide omega-3 fatty acids that help combat inflammation in the body. People who eat several weekly servings of such fish have a lower risk of Alzheimer's disease.

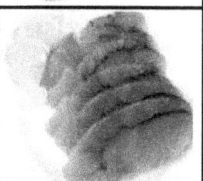

Fundamental Key # 2

Consistent exercise. There are several opinions out there as to what you should do to stay healthy. I would suggest that the real key to being healthy is being consistent. The benefits of committing to a 10-minute workout every day drastically outweighs trying to commit to doing a 30-minute workout three times per week only to actually getting to two of them because you couldn't fit it in. Doing something on a regular basis day after day, week after week, year after year is the key to lasting change. Of course, I have my suggestions on what that is as well. I have included a simple guide to help create a healthy lifestyle, this is not intended to be for weight loss, body shaping or any other therapies. I would also suggest that you consult your healthcare practioner prior to performing any exercise program.

When beginning care with a new patient I start them on a daily stretch routine to get the body moving. Once they are pain free, they are encouraged to begin a cardio exercises program for 10-15 minutes, at the very least, three days per week; preferably every day. I also encourage them to do some form of resistance training such as weight training three times per week; I believe that a program like this will help improve your health and as a result, your quality of life. I have listed some sample exercise tips below.

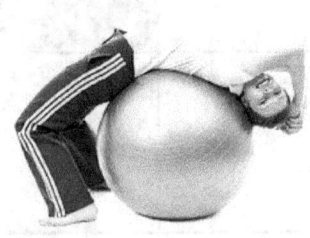

Now you have no more excuses! Here are 10 great exercises that you can do at home without the need for any equipment:

Walking – If the weather is nice, it's wonderful to get outside and enjoy the scenery around you while you exercise. However, if the weather has other ideas, you can just as easily get an effective walking workout at home. If you have a flight of stairs, go up and down them a few times. This will help to tone your legs while getting some low impact aerobic exercise as well. If you don't have any stairs available, just walk around the house a few times or you could pace while on the phone. It may not be very exciting, but it will do the job!

Jumping Jacks – These are always fun, as they bring back memories of being a kid! Who hasn't done jumping jacks for fun as a child? Well, surprise – they are also great cardio exercises and good for warming up. They benefit the lymphatic system as well.

Pushups – These are probably not the most favorite exercise for many people, but while they may be hard for most of us to do, there are modifications you can make so they are easier to do. You don't need to pretend you're Rocky and do them with one hand; just do what works for you. Do them on your knees instead of keeping your legs straight. Do them standing up against a wall or use a chair. However you do them you will be building up arm strength and muscles in your chest area.

Leg Lifts – These are great for building strength and muscle in your legs. If you find it hard to do the exercises with your legs straight, try bending them slightly.

Crunches – The best exercise for building and strengthening abdominal muscles. When you're just getting started, don't worry about getting your head all the way up. So long as you're going up until you feel the flexing of the muscles, you will see some benefit.

Jogging In Place – Jogging is a great exercise for your heart. You can jog in place at home while watching TV or listening to music.

Squats-These are wonderful exercises for your legs and buttocks. You can do squats by simply getting up and down off a chair. You can use a large fitness ball to lean on against the wall to help you perform the exercise or simply do body squats.   As long as you're able to do a few repetitions, you will provide some benefit to your body.

 Light Weight Lifting – No, you don't need to go out and buy expensive weights for this! Just use whatever you can find in your house. Start out with something lighter, such as a can of peas, and work yourself up to heavier items. You can use milk jugs, laundry detergent bottles, or even water jugs. Exercise bands are a good alternative to having clunky weights around.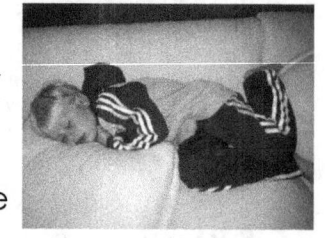

Dancing – Dancing is a wonderful exercise especially for your heart. Not only that, but it can lift your spirits as well, and give your overall mood a boost.

Step Exercises – By using the steps in your home, you can do repetitions which will tone your leg muscles.
(Just remember to be careful!)

Fundamental Key # 3

Sleep and recovery. It is suggested that you receive a full 7-8 hours of rest per night. The reason is this is the time your body does much of its repair work from both injuries and daily activities. This is when a boost to the immune system occurs. Finally, from a chiropractic perspective, this is when the discs between your vertebrae become rehydrated. This is why you feel taller when you wake up first thing in the morning. If you are misaligned and dealing with some back pain or neck pain, this is also why your back pain is much worse upon getting up in the morning.

If that is you, you may want to get an adjustment.

I commonly hear from my patients that they never get enough sleep, especially being in Silicon Valley. They either go to bed just after being on the computer or they have too much on their mind to just go to sleep. They can't just turn their mind off. I suggest that you change the focus of your mind. Here are a few tips that have seemed to help my patients.

If you are unable to get that much sleep at one time, I would highly suggest a nap. I believe a nap can do wonders for you even if it is for only 15 minutes.

Relaxing bedtime rituals to try

- Read a book or magazine by a soft light
- Take a warm bath
- Listen to soft music
- Do some easy stretches
- Wind down with a favorite hobby
- Listen to books on tape
- Make simple preparations for the next day
- Write down what's on your mind, then let it go

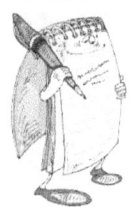

Another tip my wife and I use is a sound machine. What a great way to calm down and relax to the sound of the beach or a rain forest. I've suggested this to many of my patients and they have all been pleased. This is helpful for those who have spouses that snore!

The Harvard Women's Health Watch suggests six reasons to get enough sleep:

1. Learning and memory: Sleep helps the brain commit new information to memory through a process called memory consolidation. In studies, people who'd slept after learning a task did better on tests later.
2. Metabolism and weight: Chronic sleep deprivation may cause weight gain by affecting the way our bodies process and store carbohydrates, and by altering levels of hormones that affect our appetite.
3. Safety: Sleep debt contributes to a greater tendency to fall asleep during the daytime. These lapses may cause falls and mistakes such as medical errors, air traffic mishaps, and road accidents.
4. Mood: Sleep loss may result in irritability, impatience, inability to concentrate and moodiness. Too little sleep can also leave you too tired to do the things you like to do.
5. Cardiovascular health: Serious sleep disorders have been linked to hypertension, increased stress hormone levels and irregular heartbeat.
6. Disease: Sleep deprivation alters immune function, including the activity of the body's killer cells. Keeping up with sleep may also help fight cancer.

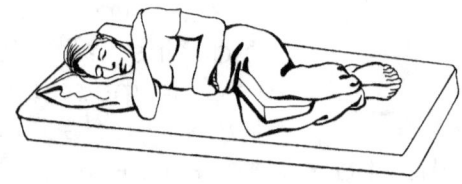

Fundamental Key # 4

Positive Mental Attitude. There have been numerous studies done on the effects of having a positive outlook on life. There have been records of miraculous cures by simply putting a person in front of funny movies for days at a time. Having a positive attitude will help drastically reduce stress which, as I mentioned earlier, is being linked as a major contributor to nearly all illnesses. If you can go through life with a choice on how you feel, why not choose to be happy. I understand there are moments that cause pain, but let's try and make these moments brief and not allow them to fester for hours or days, or worse, weeks to years. Life is too short! When I said to choose, I mean you do have a choice. It is your choice on how you are going to feel about any situation.

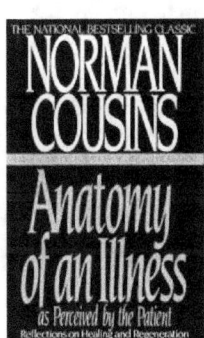

One of my favorite books is called "Anatomy of an Illness." It is written by Norman Cousins and basically discusses how he healed himself from a very devastating disease through laughter and by actively participating in his care with his doctors. I highly recommend this book to all my patients. It is a testament of how amazing your body is and what feats your body can perform, if given a chance. Attitude has a lot to do with it. There are actual physiological responses to your body, based on how you feel. To put it simply, your body can react to how you think.

"Thousands of articles in virtually all popular, medical, health and news journals tout the benefits of having a positive mental attitude on longevity and many other positive aspects of aging," says Dr. Peter Norvid, a geriatric specialist treating patients at Adventist Hinsdale and La Grange Memorial hospitals and medical director for Heartland Hospice.

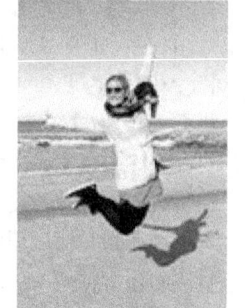

People who are optimistic live longer, have closer personal relationships and are able to deal with the negative things that happen to them in a way that allows them to continue to be able to be there for others.

Having a positive outlook helps people better cope with the challenges life brings, including dealing with the challenges of death. These people have an easier transition and allow those around them to feel more comfortable.

Having a positive mental attitude helps the body and mind 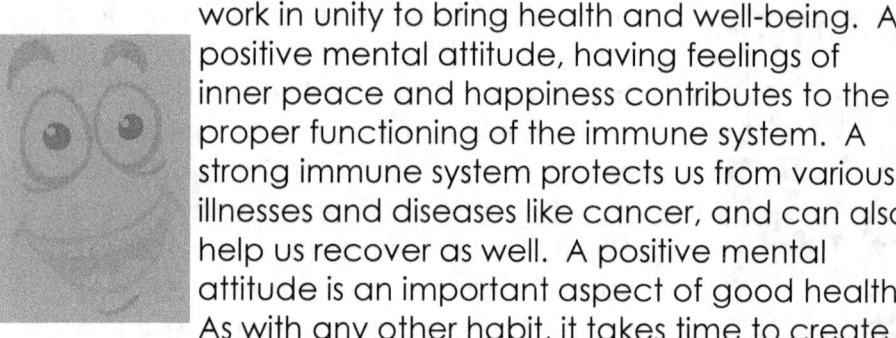 work in unity to bring health and well-being. A positive mental attitude, having feelings of inner peace and happiness contributes to the proper functioning of the immune system. A strong immune system protects us from various illnesses and diseases like cancer, and can also help us recover as well. A positive mental attitude is an important aspect of good health. As with any other habit, it takes time to create a change. As I said before, small changes done consistently over a period of time can make a significant impact. The following page contains some affirmations that may help you create a better attitude toward a specific subject. Pick one or a few and repeat them on a daily basis. Yell them out if you have to. Put emotion and feeling into it and watch things change before your eyes.

You can't have a positive life with a negative mind

EXAMPLE AFFIRMATIONS

Affirmations for health
- Every cell in my body vibrates with energy and health
- Loving myself heals my life. I nourish my mind, body and soul
- My body heals quickly and easily

Affirmations for abundance
- I prosper wherever I turn, and I know I deserve prosperity of all kinds
- The more grateful I am, the more reason I have to be grateful
- I pay my bills with love as I know abundance flows freely through me

Affirmations for weight loss
- I am the perfect weight for me
- I choose to make positive health choices for myself
- I choose to exercise regularly

Affirmations for romance
- I have a wonderful partner and we are happy and at peace
- I release any desperation and allow love to find me
- I attract only healthy relationships

Affirmations for self-esteem
- When I believe in myself, so do others
- I express my needs and feelings
- I am my own unique self; special, creative, and wonderful

Affirmations for joy and happiness
- Life is a joy filled with delightful surprises
- My life is a joy filled with love, fun and friendship.
- I choose love, joy and freedom. I open my heart and allow wonderful things to flow into my life

Fundamental Key # 5

And last, but certainly not least, a sound nervous system. The nervous system is in charge of controlling **all** functions in the body. Nothing, and I mean nothing, gets done without the nervous systems involvement. The brain communicates to the body through nerves that travel through the spinal column. So the nervous system and spinal column are very important. Any interference to the nervous system will reduce the nerve's ability to transmit information, or it will transfer the wrong information, and the nerve supply becomes compromised. Some indications of a possible nervous system interference include back pain, neck pain, radiating pain, numbness and tingling, muscle weakness, headaches and even stomach aches, to name a few.

Chronic poor posture can be an indication of possible nerve interference and is usually a result of prolonged muscle imbalances that cause weakness and an increase in tonicity in opposing muscles. Over time this can lead to loss of joint mobility in the spine, causing a segment or several segments to become fixated and irritated. This chronic irritation may become inflamed, choking the adjacent nerve and interfering with that nerve's ability to communicate properly. This can cause a host of discomforts such as local pain, radiating pain, loss of mobility and muscle aches. This condition can also have no symptoms at all, which is what makes this condition challenging. It is what chiropractors call a subluxation.

Subluxations can occur from a single incident or can develop over a lengthy period of time.

56

In the area I practice, Silicon Valley, I frequently see a patient in pain who believes their condition came on suddenly. However, after a thorough evaluation, we discover that it is a condition that has developed unnoticed over several years.

It is difficult for a patient to bridge that gap of feeling great one day then, after a seemingly innocent maneuver, sudden severe pain occurs. This sudden onset of severe pain gives the patient the illusion a quick solution can be had. That and a strong desire to get rid of this intense pain. Unfortunately, this is often not the case. It would seem that it just came on, however, after years of constant strain on the body, it could no longer handle the strain and it let go. The key is to not ignore the warning signs and get checked for subluxations by a chiropractor. The most common cause of nerve interference is a subluxation.

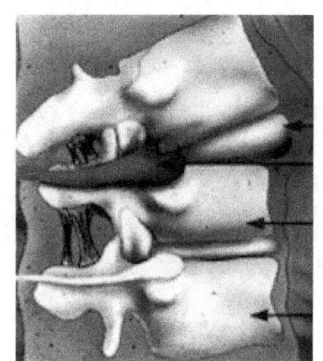

VERTEBRAL SUBLUXATION COMPLEX
(Technical Jargon)

The vertebral subluxation complex is a receptor driven compensation or mechanical adaptation to stress (physical, mental, metabolic, etc.) It is modulated by the central nervous system (CNS). Adjustments can alter the subluxation complex. In fact, the most powerful neurological treatment involving any sensory system is through the stimulation of these receptors because they involve the only pathways that bare constant active, gravitational pathways (involving muscle spindles and joint mechanoreceptors). Vision, sound and smell are turned off every day.

However, gravity is always working and constantly pulling on joint and muscle spindles to cause the creation of electronic receptor potentials. These action potentials powerfully shape the CNS and, therefore, shape all other 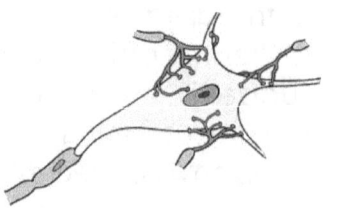 systems including the autonomic nervous system. Gravity's constant barrage of sensory information allows the adjustments to summate and change the CNS. We now know that these changes effect genetic expression or cellular immediate early gene responses (CIEGR). For gene expression to occur, the fuel for the cellular metabolism is from glucose. The promotion of aerobic respiration is from oxygen; but the activation necessary is from muscle spindles, which do not rest.

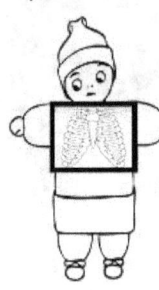 Cellular proteins must be constantly replaced in order to sustain life in the organism as well as the cell. The half-life of protein is generally 6-10 days. For proteins to remain viable, there must be CIEGR integration. Receptor potentiating is vital to this process. Adjustments not only help reduce the pain and help return an irritated segment to normalcy, they also have varying degrees of summation to the CNS.

One of my major challenges in helping a person who is dealing with a chronic condition, that has them experiencing episodes of pain that can vary in frequency and in intensity, is the difficulty of getting the patient to grasp the idea that this pain is probably a result of a very complex problem. Chronic inflammation from old nagging injuries that never healed properly contain adhesive tissues. These tissues have trapped cells causing scar tissue to develop, further hindering that segments ability to move properly.

The longer this condition is allowed to exist, the more scaring and restriction the area will be exposed to.

It isn't until a person has such a severe episode that causes them to seek emergency care where x-rays are taken that they discover they have spinal degeneration; a relentless condition that continues to progress if not attended to. This is what I am trying to help people prevent. Adjustments help prevent this!

Many people are fearful of adjustments because they believe it may hurt, or it looks and sounds like it hurts. I grew up watching Bruce Lee and a lot of his moves with an enemy's neck could look like an adjustment. No wonder people are fearful of a neck adjustment. The reality is that for most people it is a painless event. Most people get great relief from an adjustment. Initially, and depending on your situation, you may be a bit sore after an adjustment or two. But this is just old trapped inflammatory chemicals and scar tissue breaking up and freeing the area. It is similar to the pain you feel after an aggressive exercise

No amount of exercise or physical therapy can help a severely fixated segment to return to normal motion. This is why I urge people who are dealing with a chronic condition to, at the very least, consult a chiropractor.

"It is best to act with confidence, no matter how little right you
have to it."
-Lillian Hellman

Chapter 7

What is Pain?

The body speaks to us in whispers. If we don't listen, it begins to yell.
—Lisa Rankin

The International Association for the study of pain defines pain as "an unpleasant sensory and emotional experience associated with actual or potential tissue damage, or described in such terms of such damage."

Due to its complexity, pain is difficult. Not to mention the various types of pain such as sharp or dull, acute or chronic, physical and emotional, to name a few. All of these types can be just as debilitating as the next. My expertise is on the physical pain, both acute and chronic; and that is the type of pain we will be discussing.

Pain is a signal that motivates an individual to withdraw from damaging situations. A damaging situation could be a sporting event or physical activity. It can signal you that an area of the body has become weakened and is unable to keep up. A weakened condition could be doing an activity that you do on a regular basis, say, tying your shoe, and all of a sudden you have severe back pain. Both of these signals are given to protect a damaged body part while it begins to heal. If the pain is significant, it may just help you prevent similar situations in the future. Most pain resolves promptly once the painful irritation is removed and the body has a chance to recover.

Persistent pain is an indication that we have not completely healed or we have yet to remove the irritation. And sometimes pain arises in the absence of any detectable 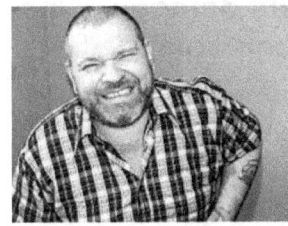 stimulus, damage or disease. Pain is the most common reason for a physician consultation in the United States.

Pain is a major symptom in many medical conditions and can significantly interfere with a person's quality of life and general functioning. Psychological factors such as social support, hypnotic suggestion, excitement or distraction can significantly modulate pain intensity or unpleasantness.

There are numerous studies that correlate chronic pain with many other illnesses or diseases such as depression, irritable bowel and fibromyalgia, to name a few. This is why I strive to find and remove the cause of the symptom thus help restore health. By restoring a person's health, you can improve one's quality of life. I may have said this before, but there is a direct correlation between health and quality of life. The type of treatment pharmaceutical companies employ consist of taking a drug to hide or remove a symptom and call it a cure. It is fool's gold. Make no mistake about it, the drugs do work in removing the symptom, but they fail to address the cause. And I have already gone into all the damages and deaths that occur on a daily basis due to what is affectionately called "side effects."

I do a half-day workshop, once per month, titled Avoid 3 Costly Mistakes Most People Make When Suffering Pain." And in that workshop one of the mistakes we discuss is the challenges that can occur when you ignore the pain signals.

.

Due to the body's efficiency, pain problems typically take years to develop before it becomes significant enough for a person to really do something about it. The problem is that by this time there may already be **permanent damage.** One day you perform the simplest of tasks, you bend over to tie your shoes and, bam, you're in pain. This is exactly what I am trying to help people avoid.

The same scenario goes for a person who gains weight through consistent poor diet choices and has ill health. Again, this process takes time. You don't usually go into a fast food restaurant to eat one greasy, fatty cheeseburger and then become obese and have a heart attack. It take years of consumption before the effects become significant. Then one day you discover you have heart disease, or worse, you have a heart attack.

Make no mistake about it, there is an effect on your body even after one poor meal; a little upset stomach here, a little indigestion there, an occasional bout of heartburn and you're on your way. I 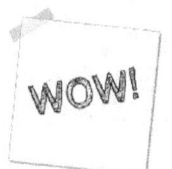 have seen what a person's blood looks like after having a fast food meal. It is literally cloudy. Your body is performing this amazing ability to adapt to these toxins every single time. This can go on for years until your body can no longer keep up.

If you continue to follow this program, do not be surprised or shocked when you find out many years from now that you are dealing with IBS, fibromyalgia, high cholesterol, diabetes or heart disease, for example. The same goes for the spine.

A little back pain here, a slight trauma there, throw in some numbness and tingling and some chronic sitting on a daily basis and you are on your way. If you continue on this path, don't be surprised to find out later that you now have a bulging disc, degenerative disc disease or degenerative joint disease.

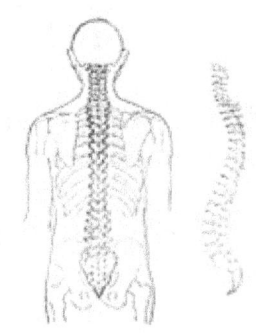

My point in all this is that we should not go on year after year ignoring the signals our body is giving us or continue to quiet the signal with harmful medications. Don't ignore the pain. And stop masking the pain.

Don't find out later on that you now have a condition that could have been prevented. Make some changes. As a chiropractor, I would suggest you get your spine checked to make sure you have no nerve interference and proper joint mobility. You will learn more about the importance of this in the next couple of chapters.

A typical patient.

Similar to the patient we talked about in the beginning of the book. I typically see patients after they have seen other healthcare practitioners and have experienced little or no success. When a patient enters my office, I begin with a thorough history. This helps me get to know the person and how this condition is affecting their life. This also helps me get an idea of how this condition may have evolved. During the history taking portion, it is common to hear that the patient has 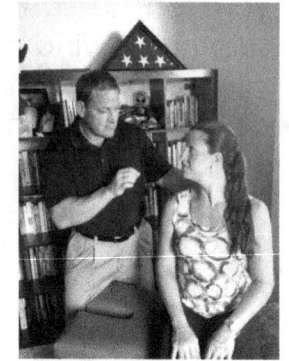 had several episodes of back pain or neck pain, or they were involved in an auto accident many years ago but, to them, it was nothing serious. They indicate that they may have had a couple of episodes of pain that even required a visit to the medical doctor's office, but this recent episode has been the most severe and is lasting the longest.

Occasionally, a patient may enter with some x-rays that 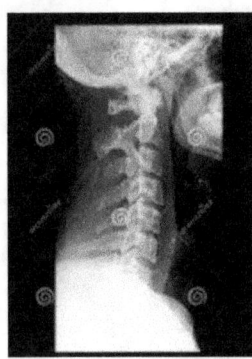 have recently been taken by their medical doctor. The doctor had explained to them that it's *just* arthritis due to "normal" aging. This quite frankly annoys me. I take a look at the films and what do you know, there is some arthritis present, some degenerative disc disease at a certain level of the cervical spine or of the lumbar spine. All the other segments of the spine appear to be normal.

If the diagnosis is degenerative disc disease or degenerative joint disease due to normal aging of the affected levels, then I ask you, how old are the rest of the joints? Were they not developed at the same time as the affected levels? Why have they not gone through the "normal" aging process?

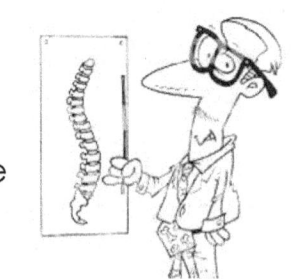

Once a complete history is performed, we begin the comprehensive examination, which includes an orthopedic evaluation, a neurological evaluation and a chiropractic evaluation. What patients often say during the examination is that this is the most complete evaluation they have ever experienced. And, sadly, I often hear the patient comment that the other doctors didn't even touch them.

After I have finished doing a complete history and a comprehensive examination, the information I gain from these exams help me determine if films are necessary. If it is necessary to take films, then we do so at that time.

Once the films are completed and I have gathered all the necessary information, I will have the patient schedule an appointment for what is called a report of findings.

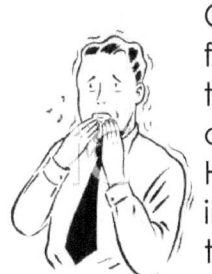

Occasionally, a patient may seem a bit frustrated that we are not beginning the treatment right away. I do understand their desire to get better as soon as possible. However, I need to take time to review all this information so that I can give this person a thorough explanation as to what I feel is causing their problems. I will also be prepared to give my suggestions on what it may take for them to get better either with my care or another healthcare professional.

I typically schedule the report of findings the following day, this gives me the time to review all the notes and evaluate the films. Once all the notes and films are reviewed, I am now prepared to give the patient their report of findings. This is one of the procedures that separates our office from other healthcare practitioners. I will sit down with the patient and explain what it is I have found and their significance with the patient. I will review with them the films so they have a clear understanding of what might be causing the pain. I will answer any of their questions. If I am able to help them, I will have some recommendations of care.

One of the comments I hear from the community is that chiropractors make you go for the rest of your life. In our office, the recommendations are given based on the individual's health care goals. What that means is that the

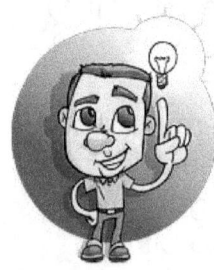

patient has a choice on how they want to proceed. If the condition is a bit more severe and I am unable to help, then I will have some suggestions on who they should go see next. Either way we will have them moving in the right direction to make some progress on their condition.

Now how often do you get to sit face to face with a doctor and really go over your condition?

I believe when dealing with some health issues, especially when it has been chronic and appears that you are not making progress, you must seek more knowledge. In my workshops I try to encourage everyone to gather all the information they can about their condition.

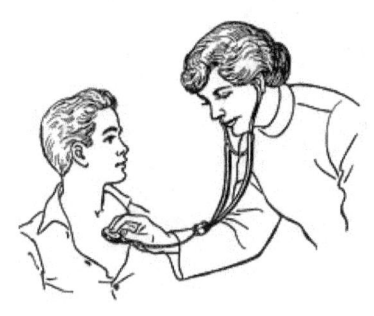

I stress that it is very important for a person who is dealing with chronic pain to "be in the know." It is imperative to gather all the facts and absorb all the knowledge you can, so that you can make an intelligent Decision. I urge everyone to not just take one expert's advise.

Unfortunately with today's healthcare, you **need** to be actively involved in your care. There is a reason you are having this symptom. Rather than simply covering it up with a pill, let's get to the cause of the symptom.

In today's healthcare system you get a prescription to mask your symptom. When that doesn't work, you receive additional testing such as blood work or some imaging. The results of those tests will determine what other drug you will need or what type of surgery will be performed. And don't expect to spend too much time with the doctor because either the insurance company won't cover the additional time or there is just too many patients to see. The further testing that is prescribed may take a while because the insurance companies need to decide if any of this testing is even necessary. Sound Familiar?

Let's look at another condition. Take blood pressure, for example. Elevated blood pressure is a symptom. If you go to the medical doctor's office, get your blood pressure taken and the marks indicate that you have high blood pressure, a really good practioner might want to get a couple of readings before prescribing you some blood pressure medicine. But there are some doctors that prescribe medications right away. So for the rest of your life you are now labeled to have high blood pressure.

Sadly, that one high reading may simply have been because you were nervous or stressed. You may have had what is called "white coat syndrome." This is when you become a little nervous and excited while visiting the doctor. This is why a good practioner would get a few readings before diagnosing you with 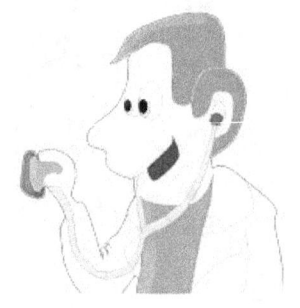 high blood pressure. The same goes for lab test results for elevated glucose or high cholesterol. Now if these results are astronomically high then you do need treatment right away.

This is why you must become more involved in your health. Do some research to see if you really need to take those drugs. Take a look at the side effects and decide for yourself if they appear to be worth it. Also, look up healthy alternatives that you may be able to employ. Re-evaluate your lifestyle, exercise routine and eating habits. I have a feeling that we could make some improvements in these areas.

If a family member of mine had a slightly elevated cholesterol level or a slightly elevated glucose on their recent blood test, I would suggest some changes and then have it tested again in 6 months. This way I can see how they are doing. For most issues, one test does not a diagnosis make.

The healthcare profession today does nothing to empower you to get better. Their idea of wellness is get your regular exams and mammograms and stay on your prescription program. They simply rely on the drugs to "cure" you. I'm sorry, it is not a cure. And taking a prescription drug to mask a symptom is NOT healthcare.

The concept of going through life as you age and begin developing these conditions that is believed to *require* prescription drugs for the rest of your life is ludicrous. Then in a few years you get to add to your routine and begin to take prescription drugs for all the side effects from the original drugs prescribed. This is why the current state of our health is poor and the average senior citizen in their "golden years" are on anywhere from 6 to 15 different prescriptions.

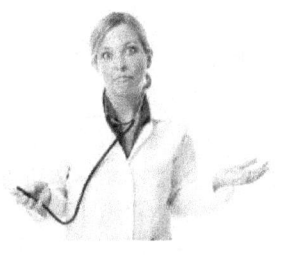

The sad truth is the medical profession has no idea what multiple prescription drugs can do to a person's body. It is appalling. Start reading and researching and empowering yourself. Learn about ways to take better care of yourself.

Based on my experience with my patients they are advised to take several prescriptions for the elevated marks after a single blood test. There is rarely a suggestion on what a patient can do to improve their marks naturally. Why? Because medical schools do not teach proper nutrition! In fact, they receive absolutely no education on nutrition! Their skill is in pharmacology. Now, I know several medical doctors who have educated themselves on proper nutrition and there are dieticians available who can make recommendations. However, for the most part, this is not the norm.

Prescription drugs continue to grow in sales and volume every single year. I have had several patients on 12 or more prescriptions! If the drugs were so effective in "curing" people of their condition, then you would think, with the extensive growth of the pharmaceutical industry, that there would be a reduction in all these conditions. The truth is more and more people every year are dying from these conditions and they continue to rise at an alarming rate. **Nobody is getting better health through life long prescription drugs.**

This system is not working, and it is not healthcare!

Now there are those patients who are not willing to do what is necessary to improve their marks and, therefore, they must take the medications. But that is their choice; isn't it?

Several of my patients enter my office after meeting with their medical doctor to go over their lab work. They are upset by the results because they are now "diabetic," or officially have "high blood pressure" or "high cholesterol." What I will suggest is that we sit down together, go over the results, and then I will give some suggestions on what they can do to improve their health without the use of these harmful drugs.

Now, let me make a note here. Prescription drugs are not within my scope of practice, and I cannot tell you to stop taking a prescribed drug and If your marks are drastically high, or chronically high threatening your health, then you may well need to take medications; but it may not have to be for a lifetime!

A few modifications in your eating habits, implementing some exercises and having a knowledgeable healthcare professional guide you, you can improve your health and quality of life. One last note: Your body is truly amazing and has the ability to heal itself. You were born to be healthy. You were given this amazing power called **innate intelligence.** This Innate intelligence knows exactly what to do.

Enthusiasm can achieve in one day what it takes centuries to achieve by reason.

Chapter 8

The Workplace

"It's not enough that we do our best; sometimes we have to do what's required."
—Sir Winston Churchill

The most unassuming culprit to back problems today is sitting. In fact, sitting in front of a computer or working on our devices such as tablets or phones is placing a tremendous amount of stress on our entire spines. Sitting is 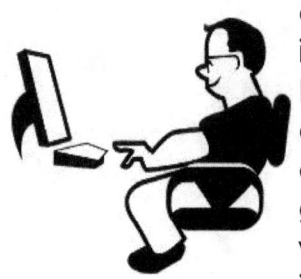 considered the new smoking. Working in the Silicon Valley for the past 24 years, I have had the opportunity to see many changes occur. The birth of the computer industry brought about rapid growth in this area. Many other services were developed to assist this massive industry. I've seen small companies grow from 3-4 people to over 100 employees in only a few months.

These once small companies are now faced with other challenges such as insurance claims and costs, loss of production due to injuries, workers compensation costs and trying to enhance this working environment that is rapidly changing. My mentor, David Vik, D.C., found a niche working with Zappos, helping them create one of the most well known workplace cultures. At one point, with his support, Zappos was considered the best place in the world to work.

The culture they created with his efforts earned him the title The Culture King. The rapid growth of culture and business changes came at a cost to the individual by way of medical problems such as carpal tunnel; neck pain; back pain; numbness and tingling in the arms, legs or both; 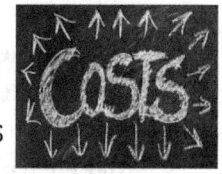 headaches and disc problems in the neck or lower back.

It was determined that the action of sitting in a chair at the desk staring at the computer all day caused these injuries. A new condition developed called repetitive stress injuries. This new condition became so costly, the companies had to seek help. Along came ergonomics.

Other than being very expensive, ergonomics' major challenge is trying to make the best of a bad situation. The task of trying to support the spine while being held for hours in a stationary position is a very difficult task. The spine is a structure that is designed to move. When you alter the natural use of any object, there are consequences. Ergonomics helps reduce the consequences, but it does not remove them. I only tell you this because I do not want people to get the impression that once they have their

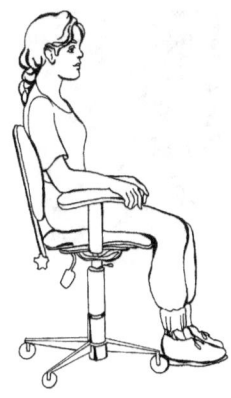 workplace evaluated and ergonomically correct, everything is ok. Sitting all day hurts the spine regardless of how well your chair is made and/or the position of your monitor or device. The information on stationary positioning and its effect on the body is constantly being updated since these injuries are a relatively new phenomenon.

This sedentary condition causes an alteration in normal biomechanics which in turn cause stress to the surrounding soft tissue structures which may become Inflamed. The inflammation may cause a choking of the surrounding nerves causing the numbness, tingling and/or muscle weakness. 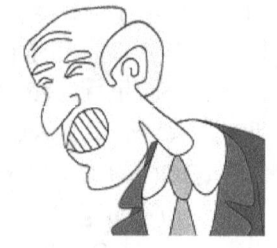 If the stressor is continued day in and day out, then the condition may become chronic. As the condition progresses you will have variations in pain and discomfort. Some people have no pain or symptoms until one day they make a simple move and then they are in significant pain and can't understand what happened.

So what is going on? While you are placing stress on the body, the body is doing all it can to adapt to that stress. The reason everyone responds differently is that there are so many factors involved in the process. How much stress is being applied? How strong is the body? Is the body being supplied with the appropriate nutrients? Is the body rested? The key point to know is as the body is adapting to the stress, you may not be aware of any injury. But if you persist to stress the body, it will eventually let you know that it needs help by creating pain. This pain is a signal letting you know that the situation needs to be addressed. Not just mask the pain with medications. Masking the signal/pain allows the condition to get worse. And over time becomes a more serious and advanced problem. It is estimated that degenerative changes to the spine can occur in 7 years. So what's my point?

Nowadays there is attention given to getting massages, sitting on a ball and incorporating core exercise which are all improvements and very helpful. Additionally, more and more people are switching to a sit-stand station, which is also an improvement.

But we can do better.

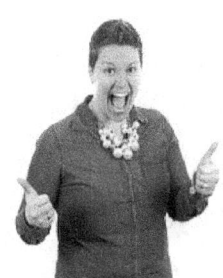

Over the years I have seem many patients that have sustained injuries to the spine, either in the neck or in the lower back. A short list includes: forward head posture; degenerative disc disease or degenerative joint disease in both the neck and lower back; carpal tunnel; muscle numbness; tingling or weakness and headaches. I have spent the last 13 years helping people remove these pains, restore normal biomechanics and improving strength to create stability in the spine. During this time with my patients, I have discovered some techniques and equipment that seems to be more effective in reducing these condition and returning a person to health.

Before we discuss what you can do to help reduce the chances of sustaining these injuries, let's talk a bit about what might be going on. Now I can write a whole book on the progression of disease in a stressed area of the spine due to repetitive stress injuries, but here is a simple explanation: The two areas of the spine that are most commonly affected are the lower cervical spine and the lower lumbar spine. It is in these areas that we generally see the beginning of spinal degeneration often due to poor biomechanics of forward head posture and/or prolonged sitting.

We need to understand that this sedentary positioning is putting stress on the spine and can continue to progress without us realizing it. This is why we need to make some modifications to what we are doing to prevent any of this chronic stress to become a permanent condition.

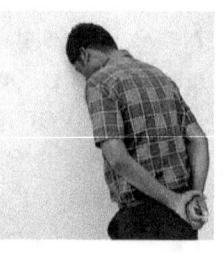

Outside the obvious such as diet, exercise and proper rest, all of which are part of the 5 fundamental keys discussed earlier, we will go over some things that can be implemented to further protect you from the potential progression of these diseases. It is my hope that you can use some of the tips in this book to help restore motion and create a more balanced body. However, it would be most beneficial for you to be evaluated by a chiropractor maybe one who focuses on restoring motion or one that specializes in proper biomechanics before starting any new routine. You want to be sure that you are implementing the appropriate exercises at the appropriate time so as not to cause more damage or pain to the tissues.

There's this notion that once you go to chiropractor you have to go forever. I am not sure where this started, but getting care is always your choice. If the chiropractor tries to hard sell you on a plan that you are not comfortable with, simply leave and go to another chiropractor.

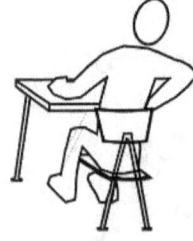

I mentioned earlier about how the body attempts to adapt to the daily stresses until it can no longer keep up. Once the body can no longer keep up, this is when disease occurs.

Don't let that happen to you.

Chapter 9

Why Chiropractic?

Keep going until you get the results you want!

With the ongoing misconceptions of chiropractic I have struggled with writing this chapter. There are those who believe chiropractic to be quackery. So, do I go technical to appease those with some medical background, or do I follow the old K.I.S.S principle. As I am sure you have gathered by now, my faith in our "healthcare" system is less than enthusiastic. Therefore I chose to **K**eep **I**t **S**uper **S**imple.

D.D. PALMER
DISCOVERER OF CHIROPRACTIC

The history of chiropractic begins a few years prior to it's discovery in 1895, by a man named Daniel David Palmer. Prior to discovering chiropractic, Dr. Palmer was very intrigued by the healing arts and how the body functions. At the time, he was a magnetic healer. He believed that getting to the root cause of a condition would be much more effective than just relieving the symptoms. This argument still exists today. Dr. Palmer felt, that all problems, such as disease or illness, come from a persons inability to fend off the invader. Dr. Palmer was intrigued when he noticed that while in a public

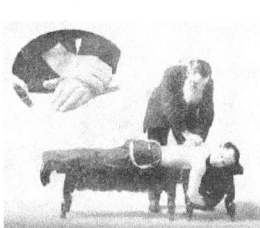

setting, several people would be exposed to the same illness yet only a small portion of those people would actually get sick. Why? What was it that did not allow those people to get the illness?

This was the basis for his research. After several years of research, came to the conclusion that interference to the nervous system reduced the body's ability to function at an optimal level, this left the body susceptible to disease and illnesses.

History states that the very first adjustment to restore nerve flow was delivered to a janitor who had been deaf his whole life. Once the adjustment was delivered and nerve flow was restored, the janitor's hearing was restored. Over 120 years 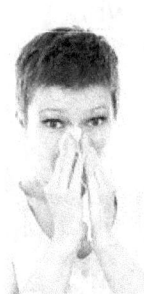 later and after years and years of research, the original premise holds true today. In fact, there was a recent study done regarding high blood pressure. To make a long story short, those who received an adjustment showed systolic and diastolic measurements drop an average of 10mmhg. This means that if your blood pressure marks were 160/95 then your marks may be reduced to 150/85.

Another study showed patients having a boost in their immune system following an adjustment. This is why I encourage my patients to come in and get adjusted when they are not feeling well.

Over the years there has been much debate on the validity of an adjustment. The American Medical Association believes chiropractic to be pseudoscience. Chiropractic gained notoriety during the early 1900s when the great flu pandemic occurred killing nearly 50-100 million people. It was one of the deadliest natural disasters. History states that if you went to the medical doctor and he discovered that you had the flu, he would simply suggest you get your things in order; there is no cure. How scary.

However, there were those who, out of desperation decided to see a chiropractor. It is believed that 75% of those who sought chiropractic care survived the deadly flu. It's funny there are people today that still see a chiropractor only out of desperation.

The medical profession states that chiropractic is not based on "solid science." Yet the "gold standard" in evaluation of potentially dangerous drugs before they get to the market is all based on the drug's ability to outperform a sugar pill. That's considered "solid science."

To put it simply, Back or neck pain is much more than a symptom. The medical profession fails to realize this. If there is no glaring issue with your films or MRI, then they really do not know what to do with your pain. They may give you a prescription of a harmful medication, or they may send you off to the physical therapist. Chiropractors evaluate and determine if you, in fact, have

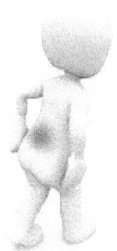

what is called a "subluxation." A subluxation is a misaligned vertebrae that is causing pain and possible nerve interference. This may be contributing to your acute pain or chronic condition. A chronic condition may be exposing your spine to what I call **pre-degenerative disc disease**. Unfortunately, it isn't until you present with the degeneration that the medical profession may have some type of care. At this point it may be injections or spinal surgery.

Once a chiropractor detects a subluxation, a course of care is prescribed based on the severity of your condition and your health care goals, all in an effort to restore health and prevent future problems such as spinal degeneration.

No other profession can do this.

Through the history of chiropractic there have been many cases of "miracle" adjustments. And there has been extensive research on the efficacy of an adjustment. Today, chiropractic is the leading choice in alternative care. Through the years there have been developments in a variety of techniques and philosophies. In the next chapter we will discuss what makes McCauley Chiropractic different.

"Serving others is one of life's most awesome
privileges."
-Albert Schweitzer

Chapter 10

Why McCauley Chiropractic?

Your body can do anything! It's your brain you have to convince.

I have been to a few doctor appointments, mostly as
support for a friend or family member,
and I am uncomfortable with the
typical treatment a patient receives.
You walk in at your scheduled time,
and the first thing you notice is that the
place is packed with very unhappy,
sick people, including the receptionist.
You are lucky if she even knows who you are. She usually just
tells you to sign in and have a seat. Now I have to decide
who is the least ill person to sit next to. Then 30 to 50 minutes
after the scheduled appointment time, you finally get to see
the doctor. The appointment then consists of a few minutes
of minimal questioning and then a prescription is given or
further testing is prescribed. I sat in a waiting room full of sick
people for nearly an hour for a five-minute visit to get a
prescription! The real tragedy is that we have all come to
accept this behavior.

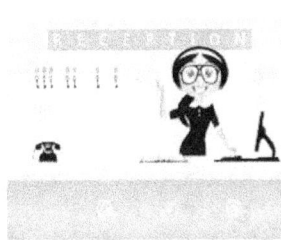

I hear these horror stories every day.
Recently, I had a patient dealing with
severe knee pain that would not seem to
go away. She explained to me that she
had been to a couple of medical doctors
who prescribed some medications and
physical therapy, but got absolutely no
relief.

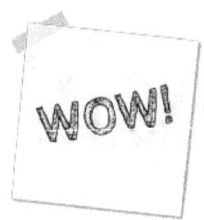

With no progress in her care, she decided to see another doctor, who took one look at her and told her she had arthritis and gave her a prescription. He made the diagnosis with a simple glance. Amazing!

This care that we've come to accept consisting of a rude receptionist, appointment times that amount to long waits and minimal treatment time and attention from the doctor is not what I would call care at all. However, it has inspired me to drastically improve the treatment of patients in my office.

The first thing that makes McCauley Chiropractic different than many other healthcare facilities in the area is that it is our policy to make the office somewhat of an escape from the stressful world. When you enter the office at McCauley Chiropractic, you receive a warm greeting from a very pleasant receptionist who already knows your name.

Our goal is to exceed your expectations. We want you to not only feel great physically, but emotionally as well. Every room has an upbeat motivational message to inspire you. Although there is an area to sit for a minute or two, we do not consider it a waiting room. Your appointment time is your appointment time. We respect your time.

As I said earlier, I have designed my office to be like a place to escape; the place where you have no worries, no stress and no confrontation.

You are seen on time and efficiently. The office is very organized. And we try to resolve any issues quickly. We explain all our procedures as we go along, so there are no surprises.

Many patients have never been to a chiropractor and frankly are not sure what it is we do. So on the initial visit, we offer a no-cost consultation.

This gives us an opportunity to get to know each other and to see if we can help. If after the consultation you decide to proceed, we begin with a thorough history. Once we gather all that information, we will perform a very detailed and comprehensive examination.

The majority of our patients state that they have never had such a detailed exam. Your history, examination and healthcare goals will determine if films are necessary. After the comprehensive initial visit, we will schedule you for your report of findings to go over all the information in detail with you and your spouse, if you choose. This gives you the ability to make an informed decision. Once the doctor has had the opportunity to review all the notes and x-rays, he will, at the report of findings, be able to let you know if, in fact, we can help. If we are unable to help you, we will direct you to the appropriate practioner. If we are able to assist you, we will have some options of care for you to consider, depending on your desired outcome. Either way, we will make some progress in your condition. If you are a candidate for chiropractic care, I will explain what it is I believe is causing your challenges, and why I believe it got to this point. I will also explain what it is we need to do to correct it. At the end of the report of findings, a patient has a really good understanding of what might be causing their problems and what type of treatment they want to follow through with.

With each and every visit we are there to support you through your care. Along with chiropractic treatments, we incorporate many other techniques to help improve your health. These include functional exercises such as specific daily stretches, ball exercises and instructions on how to support the care you are receiving. We are here for you to succeed in achieving your desired result. Our goal with each patient is to get to the root of the problem and help them address the cause to reach a point of completion.

Difference between medical office and a chiropractic office

Chiropractic Office	Medical Office
• Increase energy	• Low energy
• Friendly staff	• Unfriendly staff
• Comfortable	• Uncomfortable
• Seen on time	• Never seen on time
• Hands on	• Barely looked at
• Address the cause	• Never addresses the cause
• Explains everything	• Offers a drug
	• Does more test

Same condition, different care! Which would you choose?

Chapter 11

The Science

"In a time of deceit, telling the truth is a revolutionary act."
—George Orwell

Before we begin, I want to say that there are many different techniques used in chiropractic and all of them have their benefits. I am going to discuss the techniques we use in our practice. For the most part, we use The Palmer Method which includes diversified techniques along with a mix of activator and biomechanics from Pettibon. The Pettibon technique focuses on restoring the natural ideal curves of the spine to promote proper biomechanics. Proper biomechanics allows your body to move with the least amount of stress. Having less stress on the body helps it function at its best. With

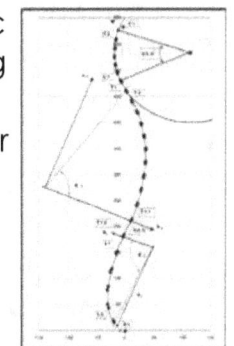

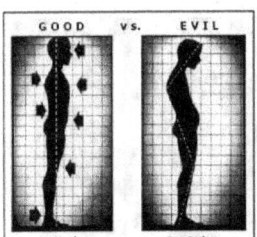

proper biomechanics and ideal curves, there is less likelihood of having any nerve interference which can prevent premature deterioration of spinal joints and the spinal disc. Poor biomechanics, or loss of curvature, causes undue stress to spinal segments and surrounding nerves, resulting in pain and premature degenerative changes. These spinal segments that have become misaligned are what we call subluxations.

There are two primary challenges to a subluxation. First, a subluxation may cause inflammation that may interfere with surrounding structures, such as the local nerve.

The irritated nerve may become painful or, worse, lose its ability to communicate properly. For example, most commonly seen nerve pain is sciatic pain. Second, and less notable, but more important, is if a particular nerve supplies your kidneys and has interference, then your kidneys are functioning less than optimally.

As mentioned previously, your nervous system controls and coordinates everything in your body. Any interference to this

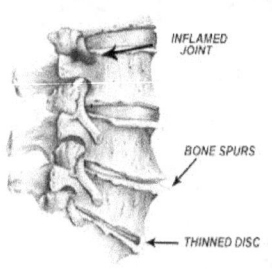

system causes that system to malfunction. If this interference is allowed to perpetuate for a lengthy period of time, permanent damage or disease may occur. A subluxation or malfunctioning spinal segment puts stress on surrounding soft tissue structures. When this situation is allowed to continue for lengthy periods of time, the surrounding structure begins to deteriorate causing permanent damage or disease, such as degenerative disc disease or degenerative joint disease. It is my belief that these conditions could be remarkably improved, or if caught early enough, they can be prevented. Motion is the key to spinal health; physical motion and joint mobility. The adjustment induces motion to a fixated segment. This concept is looked at by the medical profession with little enthusiasm.

One of the conditions I frequently deal with is called forward head posture or FHP. This condition is affectionately called the disease of Silicon Valley due to this area being the center of the computer industry. Experts call this condition the diabetes of the spine.

Much like diabetes, if this condition is allowed to continue unchecked, it may lead to more serious illnesses such as degenerative disc disease or degenerative joint disease, which could cause loss of mobility, muscle weakness and pain. As I've said before, degenerative disc disease and degenerative joint disease are relentless in their progression.

If these conditions are allowed to continue, then you may end up having no choice but spinal surgery. I am trying to help prevent this. I have seen all types of cases that have drastically improved through chiropractic care.

I have had patients come into my office the day before they were scheduled for spinal surgery, because the fear of the surgery was so great. I have had them make a remarkable recovery, avoiding the surgery. I have also seen patients with failed back surgeries who are now left to deal with a worsened condition for the rest of their lives. I've seen what can happen to a person who chooses not to get recommended chiropractic care. Several years ago a patient entered my office with severe lower back pain with associated sciatica. His films showed a severe reduction to his normal lumbar curve. I suggested a series of treatments in an effort to restore normal biomechanics to his lumbar spine, but he only wanted relief care and came for a few treatments to get out of pain.

That same patient entered my office eight years later in severe pain and leg weakness. Updated films showed severe degenerative changes to the lumbar spine (see adjacent films). It was so severe that I was unable

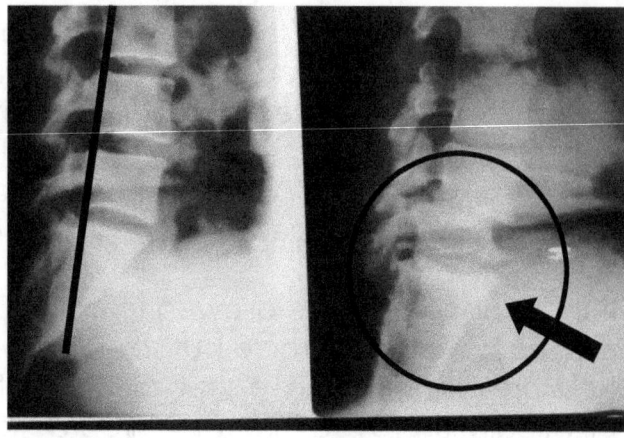

Initial film taken 8 years prior showed loss of lumbar curve.

Follow-up film shows severe damage.

to help him, I had suggested he see a spinal surgeon. This is why I urge people to take care of their condition now. Pain is a signal that something is wrong. And chronic pain is a more alarming signal.

In my workshops I urge people to get a full evaluation so that they are in the know. I want to help empower people. I want to help them gather as much information as they can, so they can make an informed decision about their situation.

Don't allow your condition to get to a point where there is permanent damage.

My goal in building this practice is to create a healthcare facility where a person feels safe and comfortable. I did not want a place that was cold and sterile, like most medical offices. I want my patients to enjoy coming to the office; and in fact, most look forward to it. I envisioned my office as a place to get away from all the stress. The stress of their job, traffic and life in general. The time a person spends in my office is all about them and what it is we can do to help support them. I want to make sure that we answer any and all questions.

An informed patient can make intelligent decisions, is empowered and is more likely to stay engaged as opposed to being a passive patient hoping the next treatment will give them relief. I have had the privilege of helping many families over the years. I've watched children grow up healthy from birth to college. I very much enjoy what I do. I am here to help.

Happiness comes when we abandon ourselves for a purpose.

Chapter 12

It takes time

Small changes done consistently over a period of time can make a huge difference.

It's a challenge helping a person who recently started to experience pain. It is more challenging when they believe that since the pain only occurred the other day and they seemingly did nothing to cause it, then it must be a simple "fix." Unfortunately, this is rarely the case. Our obsession for wanting things now, that quick fix, is actually preventing a lot of people from achieving great results and better health. You see, the medical profession gets everyone to focus on the pain, the symptom. If you alleviate the symptom, then everything is fine. The challenge with that type care is that the underlying cause of the pain was never addressed. I can assure you, as I've said before, the pain did not occur because you were deficient in aspirin or Tylenol.

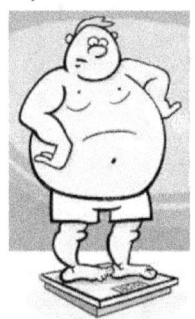

After a complete evaluation, we are usually able to find the root cause of this unexplained pain; and typically, it is due to some biomechanical changes that have developed over time. If, in fact, it is something that has been developing over several years, then it would make sense that it may take some time to truly resolve. This is similar to a person who, over several years, gradually becomes severely overweight. He or she did not eat one cheeseburger and gain 200 pounds. It took years to put the weight on, so why do we feel we can take the weight off in 30 days? It takes time to return a person back to a healthy weight.

We all know people, including ourselves, who have tried those crash diets that, after all is said and done may have enabled us to shed the pounds. Unfortunately, they are so restrictive, there is no way we can keep it up and 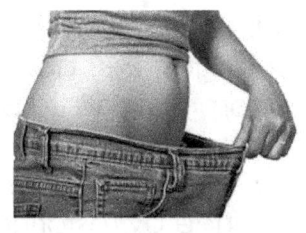 the weight, plus some, comes back. Much like embarking on a real change in eating habits and making some new healthy choices, it takes some time to see real results. The same goes when beginning an exercise program, it takes time for the body to adapt to these new stressors. But if you stay consistent and keep it up, after 12 to16 weeks, not only do you begin to see some results, but so does everyone else around you.

In my workshops I discuss the concept of a small change. I call it 1degree shift. Imagine you are taking a trip on a boat and you are heading to Europe. If at the beginning of the trip the ship was set 1degree off course, by the time you reach your destination, this ship would completely miss the whole continent! Every year in January I have several patients who attempt to get in shape or lose weight as part of their New Year's Resolution. They begin the year with excitement and enthusiasm, implementing all kinds of changes that would be beneficial; yet a few weeks later, the energy and enthusiasm is gone, and they simply get off track. This is usually because they are taking on too much or making drastic changes in a short period. Year after year they are still very overweight. If they simply made a few changes for a few weeks, then slowly add additional changes over another few weeks, by the time they reach the end of the year they have become the person they want to be.

What small changes can you make?

This whole concept of consistent changes over a period of time is incorporated into our corrective care program. To put it simply, the corrective care program is designed to create real change by restoring normal biomechanics and helping to improve posture.

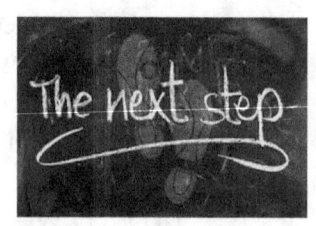

It takes time for the body to adjust to the new stressors. Not to mention the process of re-educating all the surrounding soft tissue structures that have developed a consistent pattern that a person currently holds. So with persistence over a period of time, the corrective care program can yield some significant changes.

"It takes time to succeed because success is merely the natural reward of taking time to do anything well."
-Joseph Ross

Chapter 13

Program Tips

Energy and persistence conquer all things.
–Benjamin Franklin

The following pages contain the exact information I give to my patients who are part of the Corrective Care Program. These tips are designed to help support the care being received in the office. The exercises would benefit anyone looking to make some improvements to their health. However, as I mentioned earlier, if a subluxation exists, no amount of stretches or exercises will correct it.

For my patients that are under care: These movements are described for your review. You will be instructed on when to implement each phase of the exercises. I would encourage you to wait for instruction from your chiropractor as to when to begin certain exercises, as beginning these prior to instruction may interfere or cause a setback and slow your progress.

If you have any questions about these exercises, please do not hesitate to bring them up with your doctor.

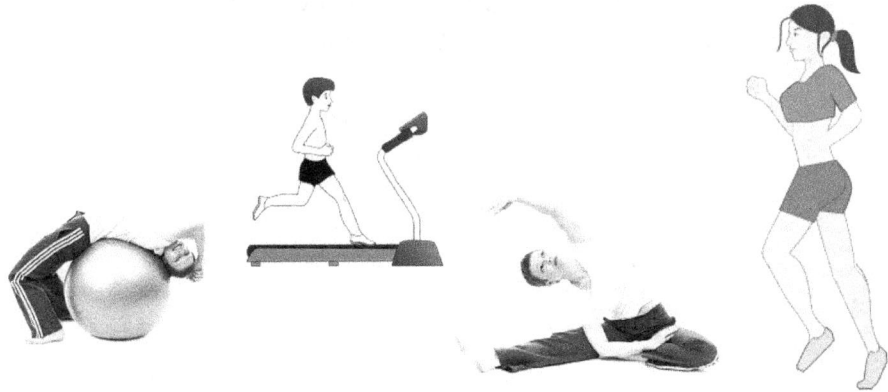

HOME CARE

DO'S AND DON'TS

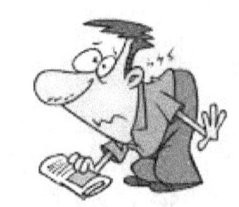

DO NOT

- Do not overextend or over flex your spine; avoid overhead work.
- Do not twist or turn your head quickly or beyond normal limits of motion.
- When lifting an object, let your legs bear the strain; hold the object as close to our body as possible and keep your back straight.
- Never bend your back to a 90-degree angle. Instead, bend your knees to minimize the strain on your lower back.
- Never sit with your legs crossed, except at the ankles. This might
  aggravate an already existing back condition.
- Try not to sleep on your stomach or raise your head off of the pillow when changing positions in bed.
- Do not sleep on more than one pillow.
- Do not read or watch TV in bed propped up on your elbows, or while lying flat on your back.
- Do not sleep sitting in a chair, with your head on the arm of a couch, or in cramped quarters.

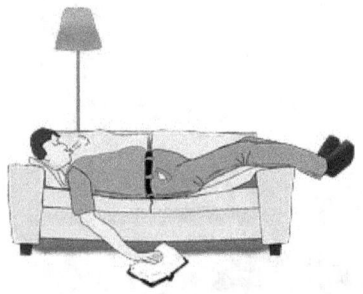

PLEASE DO

- Sit straight in a chair that has adequate firmness to hold your weight.
- Do not sit in deep, overstuffed soft chairs. Some recliner chairs are all right if the construction is such that support is provided to hold your back in a straight position.
- Be sure to get plenty of sleep to allow your body to repair and recuperate. Be sure to sleep on a firm mattress, firm enough to hold your body level after allowing the HIGH SPOTS, (shoulder and buttocks, if on your back) to fit into the mattress. If you have a waterbed, you might try putting more water into it to make it more firm. If you have severe back pain, it is better not to sleep in a waterbed for a while.
- Sleep on a pillow that keeps your neck level with the spine.
- Sleep on your back or your side. Your legs should be flexed from 30 to 45 degrees, not drawn up in a knot. When sleeping on your back, it is often helpful to place pillows under your knees so your back is flat against the bed. If you have any kind of spinal disc or low back ailment, lie down and rise from your bed from a side position, thus minimizing the amount of strain on your back.

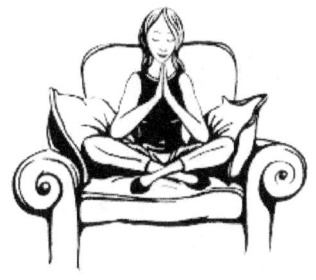 Regardless of your particular condition, set aside some special time each day for complete mental and physical relaxation, even if it is only a few minutes.

ICE OR HEAT?

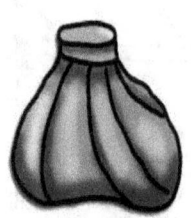

The newest therapy for musculoskeletal injuries is ice. If ice is applied to the area of joint pain, there is often a reduction of pain, swelling and muscle spasm. The cold pack should be used for only 15 to 30 minutes at a time then removed to allow the skin to warm up. If pain is felt, STOP using the ice. This is important in both the restoration and maintenance of normal health levels.

EXERCISE AND NUTRITION

Exercise should only be started when your doctor feels you are ready. Some special exercise directions will be given to you. Nutrition is very important to speed your recovery. If you have injured your spine and its supportive ligaments and muscles, you have special requirements for the following vitamins and minerals.

VITAMIN C	Helps to strengthen and repair tissue.
B VITAMINS	Helps repair nerves, reduces irritability and fatigue.
CALCIUM	Necessary for muscles and ligaments.
MAGNESIUM	If low, often there is muscle spasm or cramping.

Daily Stretches

Stretching was a major part of my preparation.
–Edwin Moses

Stretching on a regular basis has many health benefits both mental and physical. Here are some of the benefits stretching provides:

- Helps improve flexibility
- Helps lengthen tight muscles for improved posture
- Increases blood, nutrients and oxygen to the muscles, which may reduce soreness
- Helps decrease the chance of injury during exercise
- Helps calm your mind and relieve stress

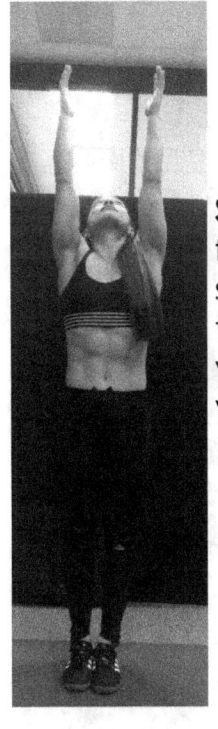

Standing Exploding Stretch: Stand with your feet hip-width distance apart, your knees soft and slightly bent, abdominal muscles tight. Take a deep breath in and extend your arms above your head, exhale bringing your arms down by your sides. Repeat 5

Standing Cat-Back Stretch: Stand with your feet hip-width apart, your knees soft and slightly bent. Gently bend forward at the waist until your hands reach your knees, use your hands on your knees for support and keep your knees soft, bending as needed for comfort. Then slowly return back to neutral position.

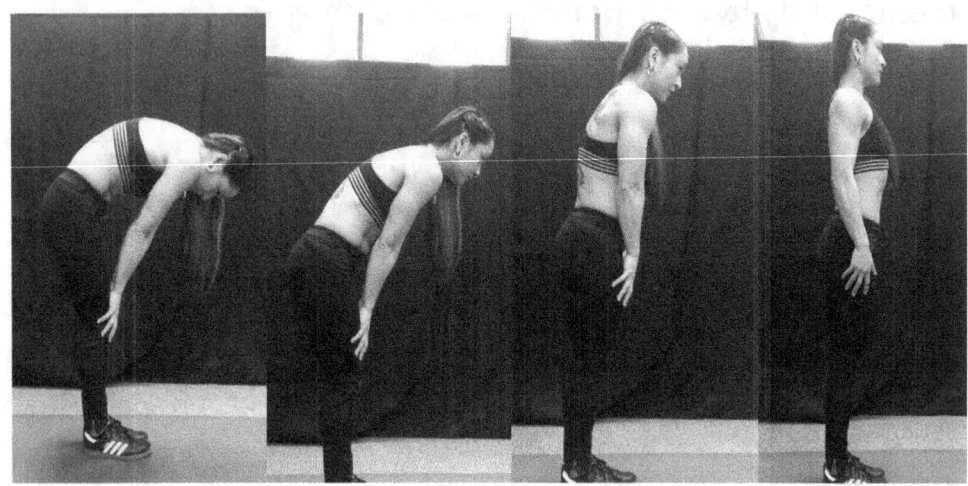

Hamstring Stretch:

I encourage you to use a chair or a counter to help with the hamstring stretch. Placing your leg up on an object as opposed to bending over or sitting on the floor seems to put less stress on the lower back. Reach for your foot while keeping your back straight and hold the position for 15 seconds. Repeat 5 times each side.

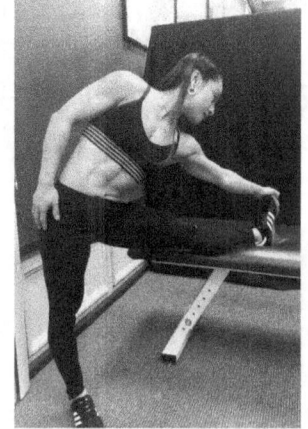

Knee to Chest: Start with both legs and feet together flat on the ground. Raise your right knee upward. And while grasping behind the knee, pull to your chest. Hold for 15 seconds, then return it to the starting position. Repeat with the other leg. Repeat 5 times with each leg, alternating between the right and left legs.

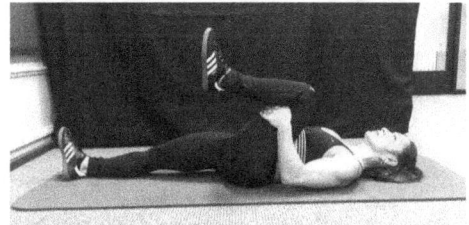

Double Knee to Chest: Start with both legs and feet together flat on the ground. Raise both knees upward. And while grasping behind the knees, pull to your chest. Hold for 15 seconds, then return it to the starting position. Repeat 5 times.

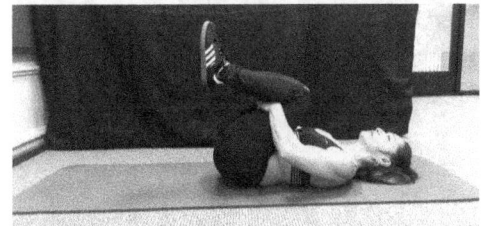

Exploding Stretch: While lying on your back on a firm surface, take a deep breath in while extending your arms above your head. Keep your stomach tight and point your toes. Exhale and bring your hands down by your side. Repeat 5 times.

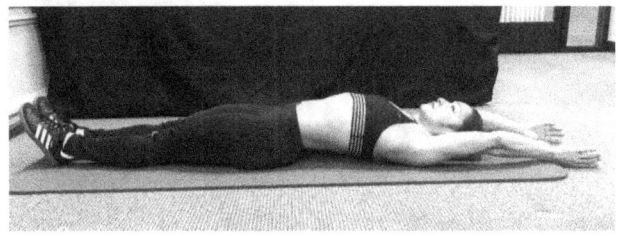

Hip Tilt: Lie on your back allowing your natural curve to occur, keeping your knees bent with your feet flat on the mat. With your arms at your side, palms flat, take a deep breath in and exhale as you lift your back up off the floor. Hold for 2 – 3 seconds. Relax and repeat 5 times.

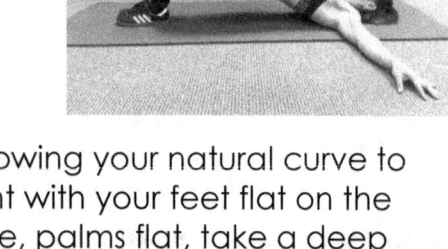

Pelvic Tilt: Lie on your back allowing your natural curve to occur, keeping your knees bent with your feet flat on the mat. With your arms at your side, palms flat, take a deep breath in and exhale as you flatten your back to the floor. Feel your spine, neck, and the back of your head pressing against the mat. Hold for 2 – 3 seconds. Relax and repeat 5 times.

Piriformis Stretch: Start with both legs and feet together flat on the ground and with both arms stretching outward at 45 degree angles away from your body. Slowly bend left knee up and let knee fall across your body to the ground to the right. Keep your shoulders as flat as possible. Hold for 15 seconds. Return to starting position. Do the same to opposite side. Repeat the exercise 5 times, alternating sides.

Lower back stretch: Start on your knees. Slowly lean forward and let your hands stretch outward and forward. Be sure to keep your head off the ground. Hold for 30 seconds. Repeat several times.

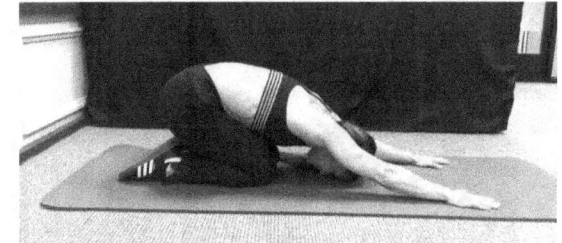

Cat back Stretch: Start in a 4–point position with your back in a neutral position. Arch back towards the ceiling, keeping the abdominal muscles tight. Hold for 10–15 seconds, then return to a neutral spine. Repeat 5 times.

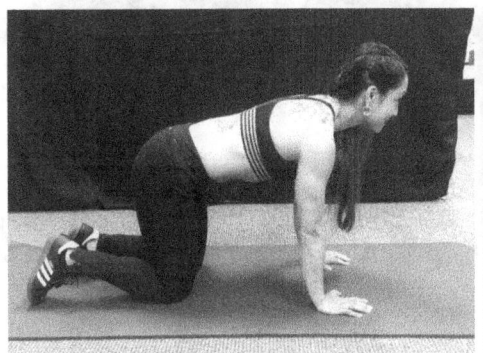 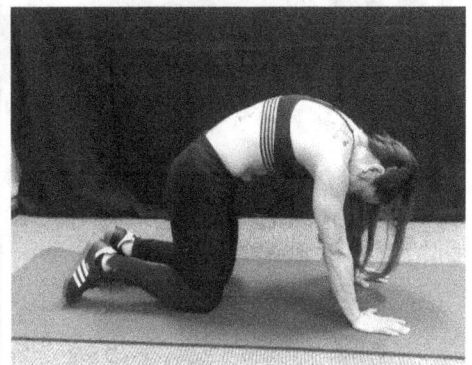

Press Up: Sphinx Position: Start by lying on your stomach. Begin to raise your upper body slowly, while keeping your pelvis flat to the floor. Try to create an arch in your low back. Go up only as far as you can without discomfort.

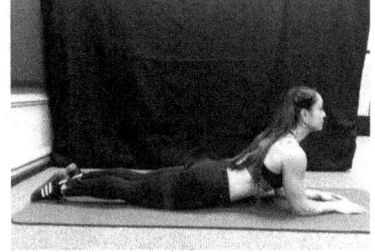

Neck stretches:

Neck Forward Flexion: Start by looking straight ahead. Slowly lower your chin toward your chest. Hold for 5 seconds, and return to starting position. 1 repetition.

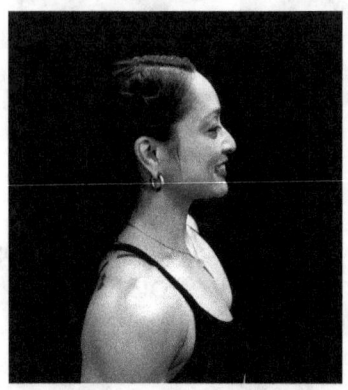 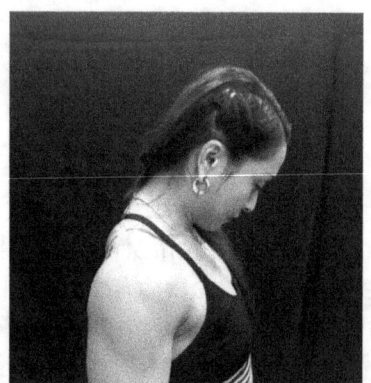

Neck Rotation: Start by looking straight ahead. Slowly turn your head to the left. Hold for ten seconds, and return to starting position. Then, slowly turn you head to the other side. 1 repetition.

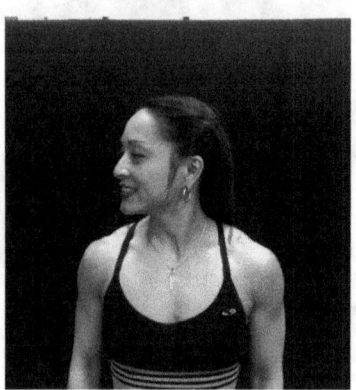 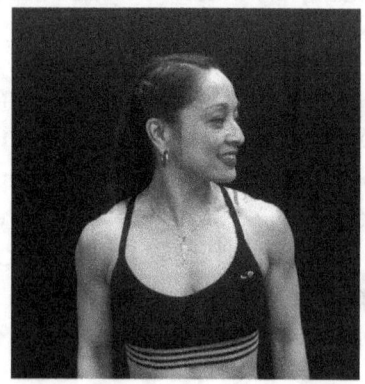

Neck Side Extension: Start by looking straight ahead. Slowly lean your head to the left. Hold for 10 seconds, and return to starting position. Then slowly lean your head to the other side. Hold for 10 seconds and return to starting position. 1 repetition.

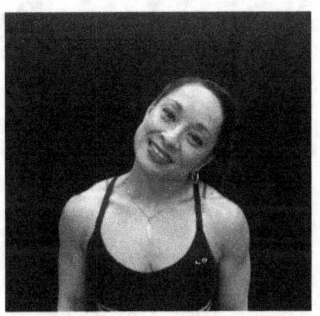 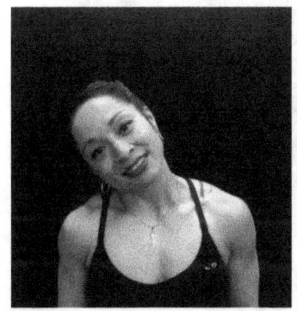

Assisted lateral Cervical Stretches: Take your middle finger of your left hand and place it on your right ear. Lightly pull your head to the side and hold for 10 seconds. Then switch sides by placing your middle finger of your right hand on your left ear. Lightly pull to the side and hold for 10 seconds. Perform this exercise in front of the mirror to help you keep your chin straight. 1 repetition.

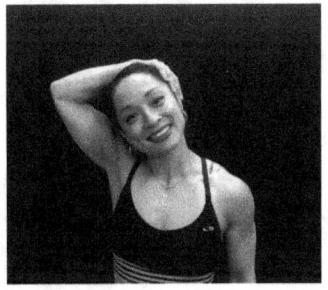 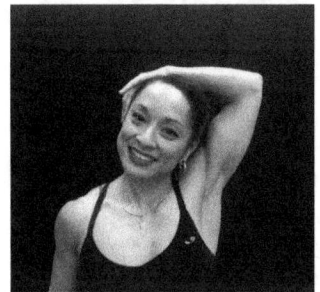

Ball Exercises

Spinal Stability Exercises on the ball
Numbers 1,2,4,5,7,9,11,12: Maintain position for a minimum of 10 seconds for 5 reps. Numbers 3,6,8,9,10: Do 3 sets of 10-30 reps or until fatigued

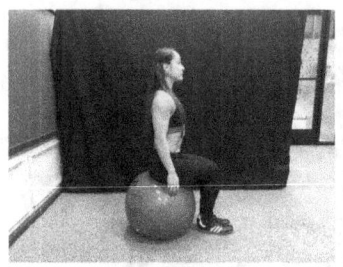

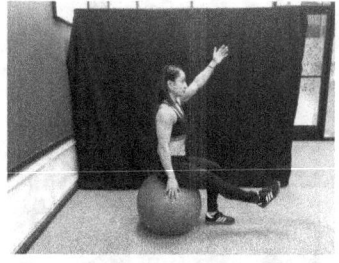

#1 Ball Sitting
Sit with feet flat in an upright posture. Keep abdominals tight, maintain lumbar curve while taking deep breaths.

#2 Ball Sitting
Copy #1, then extend one arm and opposite leg and hold for 10 sec. Repeat with opposite arm and leg.

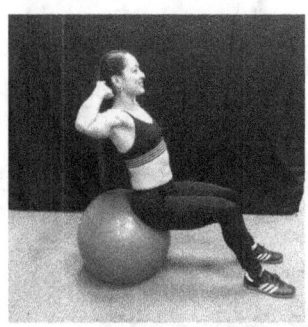

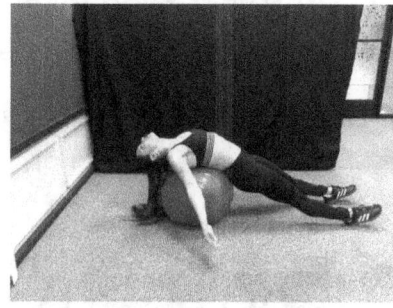

#3 Ball Crunch
With feet flat and the small of your back on the ball, perform an abdominal crunch.

#4 Back Bridge
Sit on ball, then slowly walk feet away from ball as you transition your back on to the ball.

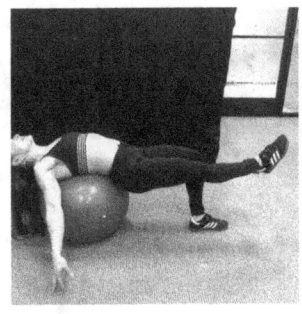

#5 Back Bridge-leg raise
While in bridge position, slowly raise one leg. Alternate legs.

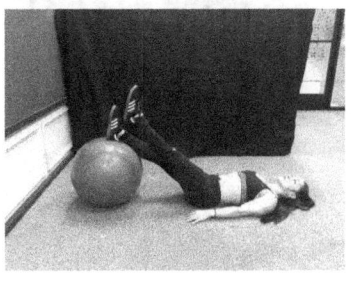

#6 Leg Circles
Lie on your back on the floor with heels on the ball. Lift one leg off ball and slowly make circles with foot. Alternate feet.

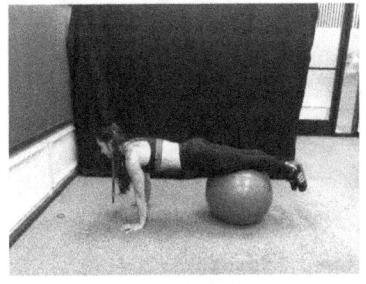

#7 Front Bridge Walk
Start with stomach on ball and hands on floor. Walk arms out until feet are on ball in a push-up position.

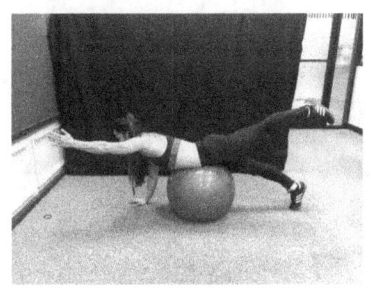

#8 Bird Dog on Ball
Lie on stomach on ball with hands and feel on floor. Extend one arm and opposite leg. Hold, then do opposite arm and leg.

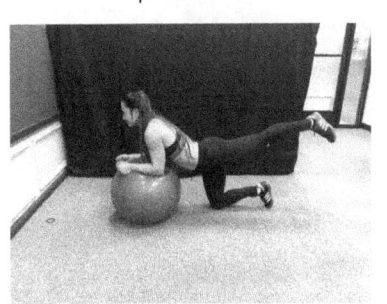

#9 Front Bridge Leg Extension
Place elbows on ball and knees on floor. Extend one leg back and hold. Repeat with opposite leg.

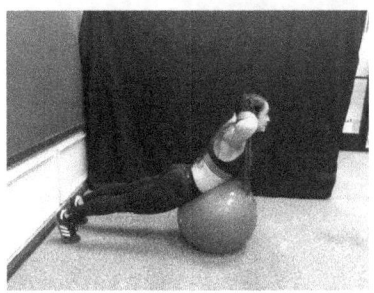

#10 Back Extension
With stomach on ball, extend torso up toward ceiling and hold. Place feet against wall for stability.

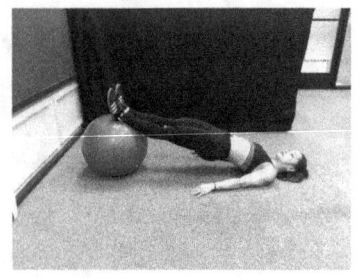 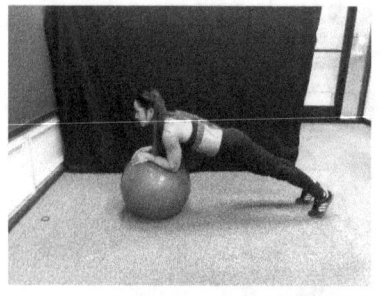

#11 Back Bridge
Lying on back with feet on ball,
raise torso off ground, keeping
your body straight.

#12 Front Bridge
Place elbows on ball and knees on
floor. Extend body off knees,
keeping your body straight.

Nothing can stop the man with the right mental attitude
from achieving his goal; nothing on earth can help the man
with the wrong mental attitude.
−Thomas Jefferson

Patients like you!

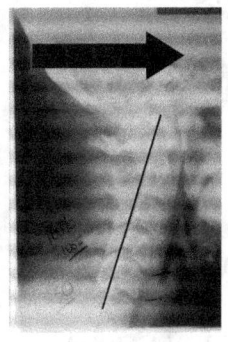

Initial X-Rays

This patient entered my office with chronic neck pain that had been present off and on for the past two years. She had been to several doctors and did some physical therapy. Nothing seemed to really get rid of the pain for good. The medication would give her some relief but only temporarily. She was getting concerned about taking so many medications. She was referred to me from another patient of mine that was very happy with her care, and she thought I could help her friend.

After a comprehensive examination and history with x-rays, we set up a course of care that would include some follow-up films to determine our progress. During the program the patient made substantial improvement. Not only did she become pain free, but she had noticed that she had become stronger during her exercises. She felt like her energy was improved which allowed her to do more. The follow-up films showed marked improvement in her spinal curvature. This improvement in both pain relief and physical stature can provide significant support for the remainder of her life!

Note on X-Rays:
Medical doctors and chiropractors look at x-rays very differently. A medical doctor is looking for fractures and gross pathologies such as tumors, degeneration of the disc or joints, congenital deformities and so on. In addition to those, our office is also interested in proper spinal alignment to support normal biomechanics.

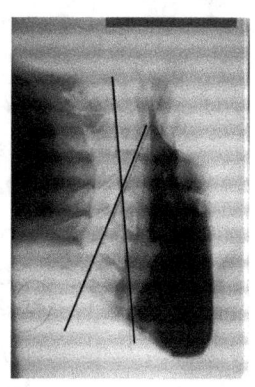

Follow-up X-Rays

Poor spinal alignment causes poor biomechanics, which irritates the affected area causing inflammation, pain, scar tissue and chronic premature degenerative changes. It has been my experience that most medical doctors would look at her initial film and consider it normal and not as a possible cause of her pain. When I look at her initial film, I see a significant loss in her normal cervical curve and moderate forward

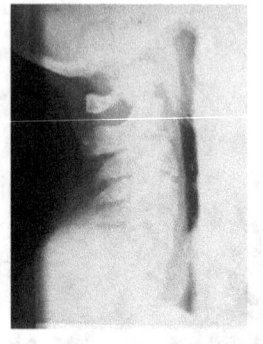

Normal View

head positioning, all of which are placing a tremendous amount of stress on her cervical spine and surrounding soft tissue structures. Over time the continued stress may cause premature degenerative changes to occur. Degenerative disc disease and degenerative joint disease are both very relentless diseases that continues to progress if left alone. I have had a patient with degeneration at one segment of her cervical spine tell me that her doctor told her that the degeneration was due to normal aging! The patient was 35 years old. This is one of many reasons why I urge people to get evaluated by a chiropractor.

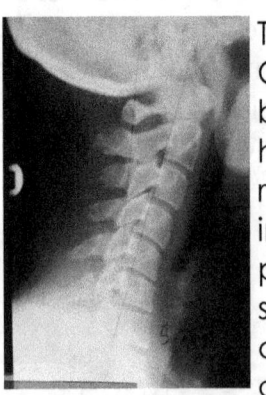

This patient is a 48- year- old male who is a CEO of a local dot com company. He has been dealing with severe neck pain and headaches for years. The pain is now radiating into his shoulders and arms interfering with his ability to perform his work. He started out with a cervical curve that was reversed and forward head posture. After a course of care, he was pain free. Plus we were able to bring his head back over the shoulders, removing the reversal of his cervical curve. This is no small task.

Medical Care:

The following are some x-rays of how the medical profession handles chronic pain that does not respond to traditional treatments.

This is what is typically done in the lower back for unresolved sciatica. The disc are removed and screws are installed.

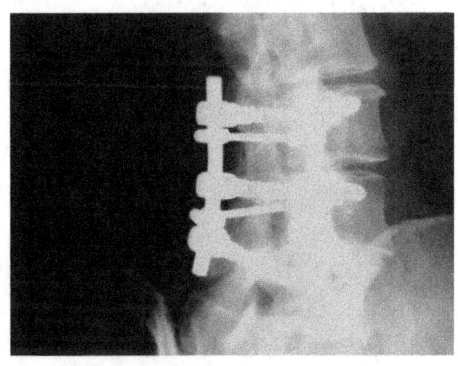

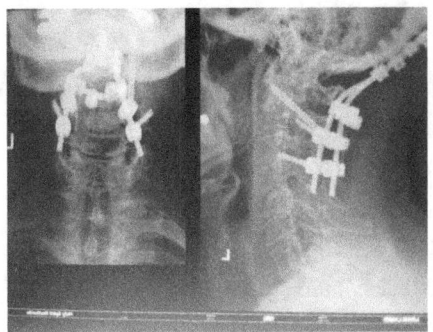

I hope this is not done very often. This patient was suffering from chronic neck pain and headaches so they screwed rods into her neck and scull. I am assuming there must have been some serious instability in there, but her daughter didn't think so.

This is what was done years ago to help with her scoliosis. This patient is now in chronic pain and can only bend at the waist.

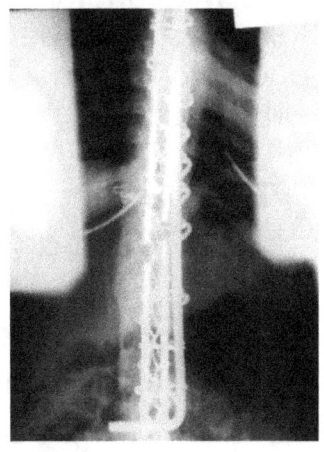

All these patients wish they hadn't done the surgery. Before any permanent procedure, why not get several opinions?

There are not many professions out there that are more rewarding than helping someone with an issue they have been dealing with for years. Working with a person over a period of time allows you to get to know them a bit more. You get to know why it is so important for this person to get back to the person they were prior to this nagging pain. After they have seen specialist after specialist telling them that their only option is drugs or surgery, the relief on a persons face when you tell them that we can help is priceless. This is why I became a chiropractor.

Chiropractic has been helping people who have not gotten the results they wanted from the medical profession for over 125 years. Yet to this day, many are still hesitant to see a chiropractor. I am hoping to change that.

I wrote this book to help reach as many people as possible, because I just may be the first voice of reason to help them improve their quality of life. I am one of many voices, but my voice, my words, came at the right time for that person to change the direction of their health for the better. If you know of anyone who is suffering and is not getting the help they need, or you are reading this and are not a patient of mine, I am offering a **free consultation**. Bring in your exams, x-rays, MRIs and any other reports you have. We will sit down, take a history, review your records, get to know each other and, if you decide you would like to move forward, then we will proceed. Let's see if I can help you.

To contact me for service or to book a speaking engagement please find me at:

my website: mccauleychiropractic.net
my email: info@mccauleychiropractic.net
my phone: 650.938.3737

Testimonials

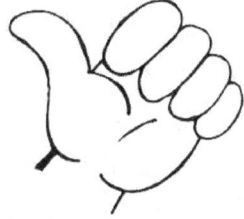

I woke up one morning with excruciating pain in my neck and had difficulty moving my right arm. Nothing seemed to help. I saw specialist after specialist and no one was able to help me. I saw a neurosurgeon who was ready to perform a surgical procedure. I had protruding discs (C4/C5).
Dr. McCauley saw me struggling in the gym for several weeks and pulled me aside to offer some advice. He knew exactly what was going on and told me that he could help. Before doing anything to me, he explained what he would be doing and what I could expect. I was skeptical but was also at the point where I was willing to try anything. Up until then nothing had worked. Sure enough, after a few appointments with Dr. McCauley, my symptoms were improving. The pain was going away and the strength in my right arm was coming back. It has been almost 5 months now that I have been seeing Dr. McCauley. I feel that I am close to 100%. I am grateful for all that he has done for me. He is passionate about what he does and for the well being of his patients. Thank you Dr. McCauley.

-JB.

Best Chiropractor in the SF Bay Area

I had been suffering from lower back pain and after seeing another chiropractor for many years and feeling like I was getting nowhere, I took the advice of a neighbor and went for a consultation with Dr. McCauley. I immediately felt I was being listened to without being rushed. It was such a pleasant consultation, free of being forced into a plan and free of being told I need adjustments for the rest of my life. What was surprisingly different was I found a Dr. that actually cared. Not for how much money he can get out of me but cared for my whole health and well being. I know I was a tough one with many ailments, but a year and a half later, Dr. McCauley has not only done an amazing job with my adjustments, he has solved some medical conditions I was suffering from that my regular Drs. failed to help me with. Dr. McCauley is honest, trustworthy, down to earth, very knowledgeable, willing to help, motivating and kind. I have gotten to know him, and I value his advice over any medical doctor I have encountered. If I had not listened to Dr. McCauley, I would have had spinal fusion surgery, knee surgery, and be on many unnecessary medications. Dr. Patrick McCauley is a chiropractor I would and do recommend to anyone who truly wants results. I am forever GRATEFUL to you, Dr. McCauley !!! Thank you for all your support.

-AC

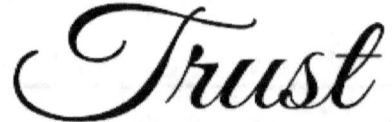

Trust

To be trusted is a greater compliment than being loved.

Back to health!

Dr. Patrick McCauley was referred to me when my back was really troubling me. He helped me through that acute stage and has kept my back and neck in good working order ever since. He is supportive and really cares. I have recommended him to others and am glad I found him!

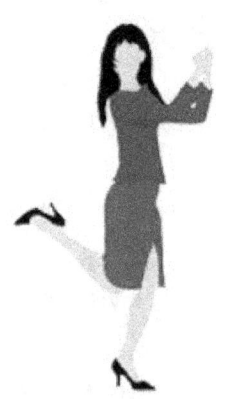

-NI

Outstanding Care

I have been a patient of Dr. McCauley for more than 10 years now. The care and service I receive from him has never been less than outstanding. He individualizes his care to meet each patient's needs and always takes time to listen. Dr. McCauley truly cares about his patients well being and it shows with every interaction. I have often joked that if he left his practice, I wouldn't go to another chiropractor. But quite honestly, I don't think I'm joking anymore....

-EH

Dr. McCauley is outstanding!

I have worked with Dr. McCauley for quite sometime. I have a degenerative disc that was causing me huge pain. I did pain meds, steroid shots and each time the pain came back and deeply affected the quality of my life. After on-going treatment with Dr. McCauley I am pain free! I have been pain free for about 5 months thus far! I can hike again, enjoy life pain free! I decided to give Dr. McCauley a raise recently as it's such a joy to be pain free thanks to his incredible healing skills.

-MK

Wonderful partner in my health care plan

Dr. McCauley is such a key player in my health care plan. I am grateful he is a part of my team. I visit weekly and know that his consistent hours and prompt attention when I arrive are key to our successful relationship. I rarely have to wait and the four long days that his office is open are helpful in fitting a visit into my busy schedule when I need to be seen. Dr. McCauley is a real professional and I have 100% confidence that my friends and family will benefit from their visits. I recommend him any time I see someone hurting. A true health advocate, Dr. McCauley always has good ideas for staying healthy and fit. Thank you for always being there when I need you most.

-KSO

What a Gift!

Six years ago I moved to the Bay Area from the East Coast. I asked my current chiropractor if he could recommend a chiropractor in my new location. He gave me Dr. McCauley's name. Little did I know at the time, what a gift that recommendation was. I could not be happier with Dr. McCauley. Consistently for 6 years I have been seeing Dr. McCauley for adjustments. Not only is he a talented chiropractor, he is also a kind person with a wonderful personality. He takes his time and gets to know you. He listens carefully to any problems you may be having and makes adjustments accordingly. I always feel better when leaving his office. My husband also goes to Dr. McCauley and is very happy too.

-DW

One of the best!

I have been going to McCauley Chiropractic for nearly 12 years, and seeing Dr. McCauley for nearly 8 of those. He is not only one of the best Doctors I know, he is one of the best people I know! He takes the time to invest in his patients, finding out about them and who they are and their lives, and doesn't just give you a 'crack' and send you on your way. He helps his patients to improve there overall health, focusing on the person as a whole. He is a very supportive and caring man. We should all be so blessed as to find someone as wonderful as Dr. McCauley!!!

-JM

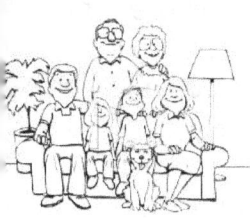

I can't wait for my Appointment

I came to Dr. McCauley with severe shoulder and neck pain. My head and neck were moving forward, and I could not straighten up, also my back was so tight. Now after several months of treatment, I am a new person; even Dr. McCauley is impressed with my progress. I still work out with weights and stretching, especially focusing on being gentler to my body. I feel more energized, can't wait for my next appointment. I am in my seventies and surely will be a patient for life. Thank you, Dr. McCauley.

-IB

Auto Accident

It is with great pleasure that I recommend Dr. McCauley. I cannot pass up an opportunity to speak of someone who has helped me live a better life! I wasn't a believer of chiropractors until I meet Dr. McCauley. After an auto accident I was referred to him for some assistance with my injuries. While being a patient I learned so much. When once I would take medications to help with pain, I now stretch and I get adjusted. I am a more complete person. Thank you Dr. McCauley for your guidance, kindness and listening skills.

-PF

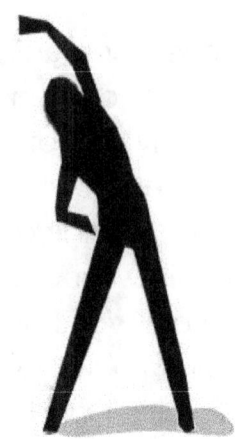

Dr. McCauley's expertise comes across with every move he makes. I'm in my seventies, but after 20 minutes with
Dr. McCauley kneading me here and there, I come out feeling much better, and a little younger because of it.

-GM

Awesome Chiropractor

Dr. McCauley is an awesome chiropractor and a wonderful man! My husband and I began seeing him 10+ years ago. We brought our 3 boys to see him 3 x weekly for years. As a result, we have all been very healthy avoiding many illnesses that have circulated throughout the years. When the boys sustained sports related injuries, Dr McCauley expedited their recovery with adjustments. I have lived in SJ for many years, and have passed many a chiropractor to get to Mountain View. It is time well spent to be treated by such an ethical, knowledgeable, and professional man. I echo JM"s review above. He takes time to invest in his patients. He cares about his patients as a whole, not just the parts of the body that need adjusting. If you want to get to the root of your ache or pain and reduce the number of medicines you take, see Dr. McCauley. He is amazing, and you too can improve your quality of life, and feel great!

-ME

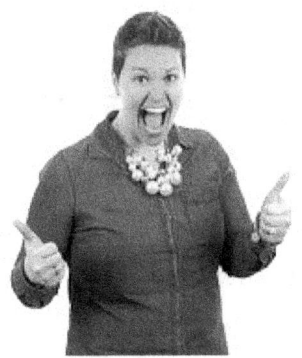

Acknowledgements

I want to take a moment and thank all the people who are so important to me and to the completion of this book.

First, I would like to thank Cindy Sauer, and Cami Peixoto for the many hours spent helping me polish this book.

I would also like to thank the fitness model Erica Ceballos for her support in providing the illustrations.

I would also like to thank Michelle Connell for taking some time to share her valued input.

I would also like to thank my children Grace and Dylan for putting up with me as I used some of "our time" to work on this book.

Last and certainly not least, I want to thank my wife Nichole who is so caring and understanding. She tends to get the brunt of my frustrations. I thank you for being so strong and understanding. I would also like to thank you for our amazing family and for making each day a wonderful day. **I love you so much!**

THANK YOU!

Support is essential to the realization of every successful outcome.
-Jeffrey Benjamin